Functional fitness for adults living with Down syndrome

functional fitness
for adults living with **Down syndrome**

Pieter-Henk Boer

WIPF *&* STOCK · Eugene, Oregon

FUNCTIONAL FITNESS FOR ADULTS LIVING WITH DOWN SYNDROME

Wipf & Stock
An Imprint of Wipf and Stock Publishers
199 W. 8th Ave., Suite 3
Eugene, OR 97401

www.wipfandstock.com

PAPERBACK ISBN: 978-1-6667-5403-2
HARDCOVER ISBN: 978-1-6667-5404-9
EBOOK ISBN: 978-1-6667-5405-6

Originally published in 2021 by AOSIS Publishing

Cover image: Photograph taken by Pieter-Henk Boer, location and date unspecified, published with permission from Pieter-Henk Boer.

The work presented in this text is dedicated to my loving brother, Rory. You define unconditional love and I am very fortunate to have you in my life.

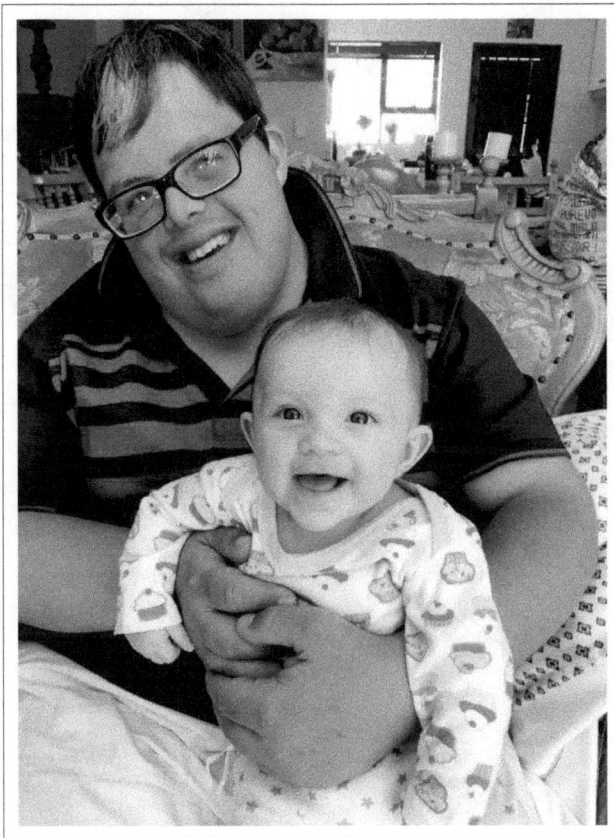

Peer review declaration

The publisher (AOSIS) endorses the South African 'National Scholarly Book Publishers Forum Best Practice for Peer Review of Scholarly Books.' The manuscript was subjected to rigorous two-step peer review prior to publication, with the identities of the reviewers not revealed to the author(s). The reviewers were independent of the publisher and/or authors in question. The reviewers commented positively on the scholarly merits of the manuscript and recommended that the manuscript be published. Where the reviewers recommended revision and/or improvements to the manuscript, the authors responded adequately to such recommendations.

Research Justification

The work presented in this book is original and represents research which has resulted from the author's post-doctoral investigations and began with his Master's and PhD work. The purpose of this book is to provide a specific group of adults living with intellectual disability (ID), namely Down syndrome (DS), their own unique instrument to assess functional fitness. Previously, individuals living with DS were pooled with individuals living with ID without DS, even though various academics and researchers have demonstrated that the presence of DS negatively affects test performance. The need arose because many adults living with DS have poor functional ability, live sedentary lives and are overweight or obese. Consequently, their quality of life decreases dramatically especially when they reach old age. This finding is evident as reported in the percentile norms (ch. 3).

Functional fitness includes parameters such as flexibility, balance, aerobic capacity, functional capacity, and muscular strength and endurance (ch. 2). The 14 test items presented in this functional fitness test battery were carefully selected after numerous literature studies and consultations with academic scholars and specialists who are experienced in working with adults living with DS. Also, extensive pilot studies were conducted in order to select test items best suited to the needs of adults living with DS. The feasibility, reliability and validity were determined specifically for adults living with DS (ch. 3). This book also provides norm- and criterion-referenced tables (ch. 3) that can be used by the academic scholar or adapted physical activity specialist to provide the adult living with DS a report card and the necessary comments or exercise prescriptions needed to maintain or improve functional fitness. Chapter 4 provides more in-depth information regarding the methodology and procedures of test administration. Chapter 5 presents information on the interpretation of test scores whilst Chapter 6 provides the academic scholar or adapted physical activity specialist with information regarding exercise prescriptions.

This scholarly book provides an economical and field-based list of test items that can be used to assess, evaluate and monitor functional fitness. The target audience is specialists in the disciplines of Sport Science, Psychological Education and Health Sciences. The book aims to contribute to the scientific discourse reflecting on the functional limitations seen in adults living with DS. The author declares that the research presented in this book is original, that the text written in this book represents a scholarly discourse, where the main target audience is research specialists working with a population of adults living with DS. Sections in this book represent a substantial reworking of two dissertations on the functional fitness capacity of adults with DS. Researches for these theses were done at Stellenbosch University and the North-West University, respectively under the supervision of Prof. Elmarie Terblanche and Prof. S.J. Moss. The reworking obtains more than 50% and the publications resulted from the theses are referred to in this book in a similar way than other referencing. These source references yield a substantial production of new knowledge and contribution to the subject matter.

Pieter-Henk Boer, Department of Human Movement Science, Faculty of Education, Cape Peninsula University of Technology, Wellington, South Africa.

Contents

Contents

Abbreviations, Appendices, Boxes, Figures and Tables Appearing in the Text and Notes

List of Abbreviations

ACSM	American College of Sports Medicine
ADL	Activities of Daily Living
ANOVA	Analysis of Variance
BMI	Body Mass Index
BOTMP	Bruininks–Oseretsky Test of Motor Proficiency
BPFT	Brockport Physical Fitness Test
DS	Down Syndrome
FFTB	Functional Fitness Test Battery
ICC	Intraclass Correlation Coefficient
ID	Intellectual Disability
MDC	Minimal Detectable Change
S&R	Chair Sit-and-Reach Test
SEM	Standard Error of Measurement
SFT	Senior Fitness Test
SMART	Specific, Measurable, Authentic, Realistic, Time
SOOL	Standing On One Leg
WOBB	Walking on Balance Beam

List of Appendices

Boxes

List of Figures

List of Tables

Biographical Note

Pieter-Henk Boer
Department of Human Movement Science,
Faculty of Education, Cape Peninsula University of Technology,
Wellington, South Africa
Email: boerpi@cput.ac.za
ORCID: https://orcid.org/0000-0003-3622-2599

Pieter-Henk Boer (PhD) is a lecturer and researcher at the Cape Peninsula University of Technology, Wellington, South Africa. He received his Master's and PhD degrees in Adapted Physical Activity, focusing on the functional fitness of adults living with Down syndrome (DS). He has authored and coauthored numerous papers regarding the functional fitness assessment and exercise prescription for adults living with DS. Dr Boer obtained his Master's in Sport Science at Stellenbosch University and his PhD in Human Movement Science at North-West University. Dr Boer is an NRF-rated researcher (Y-category). He worked for 6 years at the Department of Sport Science at the North-West University as a Senior Lecturer and Head of Department before moving to Wellington. In 2013, Dr Boer was awarded the Faculty Junior Researcher of the year award. He also achieved the teaching and learning prize for his campus in the yearly Institutional Teaching Excellence Award (ITEA). Dr Boer has a sibling living with DS and has worked extensively at Intellectual Disabled Care Centres.

Declaration

The book, entitled *Functional fitness for adults living with Down syndrome,* presents Dr Pieter-Henk Boer Masters and PhD research findings. The Masters' thesis, 'The functional fitness capacity of adults with Down syndrome in South Africa' (2010) submitted to the Department of Sport Science, Stellenbosch University. The PhD thesis, 'Effect of continuous aerobic vs interval training on selected functional fitness parameters of adults with intellectual disability and Down syndrome' (2015), was submitted to Physical Activity, Sport and Recreation, North-West University. The book represents a reworking of more than 55% of the original theses to meet the standards of the publisher and the Department of Higher Education and Training (DHET). It is his work in conception and execution, and all the relevant sources that he has used or quoted have been indicated and acknowledged by means of complete references.

Acknowledgement

Thank you to the Almighty God for providing me with the necessary skills and social support to complete the research presented herein. Thank you to my family, Chandré, Lienke-Mari, Mieke-Louise and extended family for the motivation provided during the writing of this text. I would also like to thank Luiba for providing all the pictures illustrated in this book. Lastly, I would like to thank Stellenbosch University, North-West University, Cape Peninsula University of Technology as well as my two study leaders (Prof. Terblanche and Prof. Moss) during my Master's, PhD and post PhD studies (2009–2021).

Introduction

The work presented in this book represents research which has resulted from the author's post-doctoral investigations and began with his Master's and PhD work. The purpose of this book is to provide a specific group of adults living with intellectual disability (ID), namely Down syndrome (DS), their own unique instrument to assess functional fitness. Previously, individuals living with DS were pooled with individuals living with ID without DS, even though various academics and researchers have demonstrated that the presence of DS negatively affects test performance. The need arose because many adults living with DS have poor functional ability, live sedentary lives and are overweight or obese. Consequently, their quality of life decreases dramatically especially when they reach old age. This finding is evident as reported in the percentile norms (ch. 3). Also, because of the advancements of medical technology, the life expectancy of individuals living with DS has increased vastly but is concerning because many adults living with DS age prematurely and become dependent on others at the age of 45 years. In many cases, this age-related dependency accrues at a much younger age, especially when obesity and other frequently occurring conditions such as cardiovascular or musculoskeletal problems arise.

Consequently, the goal was to develop a holistic functional fitness instrument of test items adapted to the needs of adults living with DS (18 years and older). The use of the word 'holistic' refers to all of the physical parameters indicative of functional fitness such as body mass index, balance, flexibility, musculoskeletal strength, aerobic capacity and functional ability. The 14 test items presented in this functional fitness test battery were carefully selected after numerous literature studies and consultations with academic scholars and specialists who are experienced in working with adults living with DS. Also, extensive pilot studies were conducted in order to select test items best suited to the needs of adults living with DS. Because of their poor functional fitness, it is not surprising that test items suited to the needs of other functionally impaired populations (the elderly in the general population and individuals with ID) were selected. Therefore, test items with well-established feasibility, reliability and validity were included. Furthermore, the feasibility, reliability and validity were once again determined specifically for adults living with DS (ch. 3). This book also provides norm- and criterion-referenced tables (ch. 3) that can be used by the academic scholar or adapted physical activity specialist to provide the adult living with DS a report card

How to cite: Boer, P.-H., 2021, 'Introduction', in *Functional fitness for adults living with Down syndrome*, pp. 1–2, AOSIS, Cape Town. https://doi.org/10.4102/aosis.2021.BK252.00

and the necessary comments or exercise prescriptions needed to maintain or improve functional fitness.

Subsequently, this book provides a simple, economical and field-based list of test items that can be used to assess, evaluate and monitor functional fitness. In doing so, many of the functional limitations seen in adults living with DS may be prevented or reversed before more serious physical conditions such as walking difficulties and dependency on others ensue.

Unfortunately, the tests presented in this book are not designed for those with severe ID who cannot understand test instructions or procedures or those with physical limitations contraindicative to exercise. Many individuals living with DS suffer from congenital heart disease and other clinical or physical conditions and therefore the adapted physical activity readiness questionnaire and informed consent form are attached as appendixes to this book (app. A and app. G). The primary physician of the adult living with DS must be consulted before test administration. Lastly, the tests presented in this book are not developed for adults living with mosaic type DS (1% of all DS cases) as their physical and intellectual disabilities are superior to those with trisomy type 21 DS. Although, they may participate in testing, their results should not be evaluated with the norm- and criterion-referenced tables presented in Chapter 3.

The texts provided in this book are grouped into six chapters. Chapter 1 provides an overview of functional fitness, whereas Chapter 2 provides more specific information pertaining to the functional fitness test battery for adults living with DS. As previously highlighted, Chapter 3 reports on the standardisation of test items, whilst Chapter 4 provides more in-depth information regarding the methodology and procedures of test administration. Lastly, Chapter 5 presents information on the interpretation of test scores whilst Chapter 6 provides the academic scholar or adapted physical activity specialist with information regarding exercise prescriptions. Many appendixes that are referenced throughout the book (important for test administration and interpretation) are attached.

What is functional fitness?

◼ Background

Functional fitness is defined by Rikli and Jones (2013:2) as 'having the physical capacity to perform normal everyday activities safely and independently without undue fatigue'. Millán-Calenti et al. (2010:306) provided a similar definition of functional fitness as 'having the ability to carry out daily activities in a normal and acceptable manner'. These definitions illustrate that functional fitness is instrumental for quality of life and especially it is required when we age.

Using the term 'functional fitness' rather than the more widely used 'physical fitness' is paramount as it explicitly focusses on functional capacity, ability and health as opposed to physical skill or performance as studied in athletic populations. However, it is challenging to directly measure functional fitness as it is difficult to measure or quantify one's performance in daily tasks (Reiman & Manske 2009). Fortunately, many physical factors have been identified that contribute to functional fitness (Arena et al. 2007:329; Brill 2004:5; Rikli & Jones 2013:12; Singh et al. 2006:4). Arena et al. (2007:329) demonstrated that functional fitness is associated with the ability to perform activities of daily living (ADL) that require a sustained aerobic metabolism. Specifically, these researchers referred to the integrated effort of the

How to cite: Boer, P.-H., 2021, 'What is functional fitness?', in *Functional fitness for adults living with Down syndrome*, pp. 3-14, AOSIS, Cape Town. https://doi.org/10.4102/aosis.2021.BK252.01

cardiopulmonary and skeletal muscle systems involved with functional capacity. Rikli and Jones (2013:14) and Brill (2004:5) also stated that it is imperative to determine which physical qualities are related to functional fitness. In Chapter 2, the factors associated with functional fitness will be discussed in further detail.

■ Importance of functional fitness

Most people take their health and functional fitness for granted. When one reaches old age or physical and clinical conditions or disabilities arise, one realises how important a functionally active and healthy lifestyle is. Exercise is Medicine©, a global health initiative managed by the American College of Sport Medicine (ACSM), has embarked to educate all people and health practitioners on the importance of a functionally active lifestyle (Lobelo, Stoutenberg & Hutber 2014:1627). This initiative is gaining more popularity as many people around the world are living with chronic medical conditions. More health practitioners are including exercise prescriptions or at least a referral letter to a registered exercise specialist in their treatment plans. Many people worldwide are suffering from chronic-related conditions (such as diabetes, obesity, hypertension, osteoporosis, Parkinson's and cardiovascular disease) which impair their functional fitness. The benefits of living a functionally active lifestyle and the indirect relationship between physical activity and the development of chronic conditions have been well documented (World Health Organization 2010). This finding along with the relationship between physical activity and quality of life has also been reiterated by the ACSM specifically for persons with chronic diseases or disability (Moore et al. 2016). The '[p]opulations at risk to develop low functional fitness' section will provide a brief overview of populations at risk for developing low functional fitness including those with physical and intellectual disabilities (IDs).

■ Populations at risk to develop low functional fitness

The first group of people that one could envisage as being prone to low functional fitness is the elderly.

Terblanche and Boer (2013) describe the investigation of Millán-Calenti et al. (2010:306) and Chalise, Saito and Kai (2008:394) into the 'activities of daily living (ADL) such as bathing, eating and dressing, and instrumental activities of daily living (IADL) such as housework, shopping, and gardening, in large samples of elderly adults' and emphasise the conclusion drawn by these authors that (Terblanche & Boer 2013):

[*W*]ith increasing age, health and functional status declines, physical and cognitive abilities decrease and the number of chronic diseases and the extent of disability in performing daily activities increase. Functional dependence also correlated significantly with the number of visits to the doctor, days spent in hospital, and illnesses such as dementia. (pp. 826–836)

These studies, amongst many others, demonstrate the importance of maintaining adequate functional capacity for doing daily activities successfully in old age.

Individuals with chronic physical or psychological conditions are another group with lower functional fitness. Various studies have focused on the phenomenon. Terblanche and Boer (2013) refer to clinical studies which explained that 'majority of individuals with chronic heart disease have low functional capacity' (Arena et al. 2007:333; Bocalini, Santos & Serra 2008:437). Brill (2004:31) also reported 'low functional capacity and other chronic conditions such as arthritis, diabetes, hypertension, Parkinson's disease, stroke, low back pain, osteoporosis, and those with hip fractures' (Terblanche & Boer 2013). They found that most people over the age of 65 years have at least one chronic health condition impairing functional fitness and wellbeing (see Terblanche & Boer 2013). Obesity, affecting many people worldwide has also been reported to be an independent contributor to impaired functional capacity (Oeser et al. 2005:3651; Pataky et al. 2014:56).

Another group of people who are possibly prone to lower functional fitness are the physically or intellectually disabled people. The Americans with Disabilities Act defines disability as 'a physical or mental impairment that substantially limits one or more of the major life activities'[1]. A disability can be classified as any type of disorder that limits a person's ability to perform a normal daily routine (Rimmer, Braddock & Pitetti 1996:1367). What makes these definitions unique is its significance from a functional performance perspective as it could potentially affect ADL and instrumental ADL. A sub-category of intellectually disabled individuals is those living with DS. They might be particularly susceptible to low levels of functional capacity because of poor physical fitness (Baynard et al. 2004:1285, 2008:1984; Boer 2010:105; Carmeli et al. 2004:17; Pitetti & Boneh 1995:423; Tsimaras & Fotiadou 2004:343), obesity (Terblanche & Boer 2013:830) and a sedentary lifestyle (Nordstrøm et al. 2013:4395). Specifically, these researchers found that individuals living with DS have poor aerobic capacities, poor muscular strength, poor balance, and poor functional fitness when compared to the general population or those living with an ID without DS. The 'Background of Down syndrome' section provides background information pertaining to the condition known as DS.

----

1. See Americans with Disabilities Act, Coverage of Contagious Diseases (2011).

■ Background of Down syndrome

▨ What is the condition known as Down syndrome?

Down syndrome occurs when an individual has a full or partial additional copy of the 21st chromosome. Down syndrome is the most prevailing chromosomal cause of ID (Barnhart & Connolly 2007:1399; National Down Syndrome Society 2020). The extra chromosome results in a disruption of gene expression and influences the structure and function of all physiological systems (Boer 2015:25). Down syndrome is not a disease but a genetic abnormality. It is associated with an ID that is not a sign of future limitations or functional incapacity (Boer 2015:26). Individuals living with DS have unique physical characteristics, altered development patterns, and most individuals have moderate to mild ID (National Down Syndrome Society 2020). Unlike those living with ID without DS, DS is dispersed across all socio-economic classes. In today's society, many individuals living with DS attend school, work, recreate and participate in sporting events (Boer 2015:26). There are many initiatives, such as South Africa's National Down Syndrome Society, that drive DS inclusion into everyday society. There is also an World Down Syndrome Congress held every 2-3 years to promote fundamental issues for optimal development such as sound education, stimulating environments, adequate health care and social support. Because of improved healthcare and education, most adults living with DS can hold a job or function well in a centre for the intellectually disabled (Smith 2001:1031). Many individuals living with DS function independently in the community with minimal support for most of their adult life (Smith 2001:1031).

▨ Types of Down syndrome

Down syndrome results from three likely causes that are all chromosome abnormalities. All three causes are related to a full or partial additional copy of the 21st chromosome. Trisomy 21 is the most frequent occurrence (95% of all cases) and results, as the name suggests, in an additional 21st chromosome (Mutton & Alberman 1996:387). These individuals have 47 chromosomes instead of 46 (23 from each parent). A second cause is translocation (4% of all cases) and as in trisomy 21, there is still a third 21st chromosome, but one of these grows onto another chromosome, appearing as one, but containing the genetic material of two chromosomes (Boer 2015:27). The most common occurrence being Robertsonian where chromosome 14 and 21 are involved. Lastly, a third possible form is mosaic DS (1% of all cases). These individuals have two cell lines, one of which contains 46 chromosomes and the other 47 chromosomes. These are the individuals living with DS who are most likely to attend school or university (Boer 2015:27).

Incidence and life expectancy

The number of individuals living with DS in the United States of America is approximately 250 700 and the prevalence is currently 8.27 per 10 000 (Presson et al. 2013:1163). There are no published reports on prevalence of DS in developing countries but Down Syndrome South Africa (DSSA) (2020) published findings indicating that 1 in 1000 live births in developed countries are DS and this statistic increases to 2 per 1000 in developing countries (Boer 2015:28; DSSA 2020).

The life expectancy of individuals living with DS has increased drastically over the past three decades with many individuals reaching middle to old age (Chicoine & McGuire 1997:477; Torr et al. 2010:70). Chicoine and McGuire (1997:477) reported that a woman living with DS lived up to the age of 83 in the United States of America. Specifically, Yang et al. (2002:1019) reported that the mean life expectancy has increased from 25 years in 1983 to 49 years in 1997. The mortality in individuals living with DS is the highest amongst those with congenital anomalies (Abbag 2006:219). If early intervention strategies for congenital abnormalities had been implemented, the 1-year survival increased tremendously, reaching almost 100% (Irving et al. 2008:1336). Even though life expectancy has increased in this population, it has been shown that individuals living with DS have a fundamentally different ageing process (Barnhart & Connolly 2007:1400–1401). Specifically, it has been reported that adults living with DS age prematurely (Carfi et al. 2014:51; Oliver et al. 1998:1365; Terblanche & Boer 2013:834; Torr et al. 2010:70). Consequently, the maintenance of functional fitness is of cardinal importance in a population with an ever-increasing life expectancy as ageing and the effects thereof occur prematurely.

Health, obesity and sedentary lifestyle in adults living with Down syndrome

Down syndrome individuals are born with many health-related disorders of which congenital heart disease is the most common at 61% of all cases (Abbag 2006:219; Boer 2015:29). The most common congenital heart disease reported was ventricular and atrioventricular septal defect which accounted for 56% of all cases (Abbag 2006:219). These individuals are at greater risk of developing thyroid problems, leukaemia and respiratory complications that will eventually require surgery or treatment (Boer 2015:29; De Asua et al. 2015:385; Hermon et al. 2001:167; NDSS 2020; Pikora et al. 2014:e96868; Smith 2001:1031). Yang et al. (2002:1019) demonstrated that these conditions were often the cause of mortality. Specifically, the authors stated that the most common causes of death in descending order of frequency were congenital heart disease, dementia, hypothyroidism and leukaemia. Leukaemia was the only form of cancer frequently encountered in this population with all other malignant type conditions having a strikingly low odds ratio. The authors explained that this could be because of a decreased exposure to environmental factors, tumour-suppressing genes on chromosome 21 or a slower rate of replication of cancerous cells.

Adults living with DS are also at a greater risk of developing diabetes, Alzheimer's disease, depression, obsessive-compulsive disorder, epilepsy and mitochondrial dysfunction (Boer 2015:29; Hermon et al. 2001:167; Izzo et al. 2018). Torr et al. (2010:70) have reiterated that dementia of the Alzheimer's type was highly prevalent in this population and especially in the sixth decade of life. In all these conditions, behavioural changes or loss of a function may be the only signs of the disease (Smith 2001:1031).

A large percentage of individuals living with DS are overweight or obese (Boer 2015:30; Carmeli et al. 2002:460; Melville et al. 2008:425; Pitetti, Baynard & Agiovlasitis 2013:47; Prasher & Filer 1995:437; Rubin et al. 1998:175; Terblanche & Boer 2013:830). Rubin et al. (1998:178) demonstrated that 45% of men and 56% of women are overweight whilst Terblanche and Boer (2013:830) found that 79% of men and 95% of women are overweight in a sample of 371 individuals living with DS in South Africa. It may not be appropriate to use body mass index (BMI) as an indication of obesity in this population because of their inherent short stature. However, a study by Baptista, Varela and Sardinha (2005:382) indicated a higher body fat mass in this population compared to the general population. Furthermore, individuals living with DS have an increased risk of obesity compared to individuals living with ID without DS (Melville et al. 2008:425). Rubin et al. (1998:175) reported that individuals living with DS residing in a private home had a greater tendency to be overweight compared to those living communally. One of the causes may be easier access to food. Being overweight is a risk factor for cardiovascular disease and could act as a mediator to develop other chronic conditions in this population (Rubin et al. 1998:179). Obesity has been associated with hypertension, diabetes, premature ageing and other health-related diseases in the general population (Boer 2015:31; Chiang, Pritchard & Nagy 2011:700; Iacobellis et al. 2005:1116; Niemann et al. 2011:577). It is uncertain whether the same association is found in the DS population.

Unfortunately, most individuals living with DS have sedentary lifestyles (Boer 2015:31; Esposito et al. 2012:109; Nordstrøm et al. 2013:4395; Shields, Dodd & Abblitt 2009:307). Only 42% of children living with DS performed at least 60 min of moderate to vigorous exercise per day (Shields et al. 2009:307). A study in Norway showed that only 12% of individuals living with DS, Prader-Willi syndrome and Williams syndrome (18–45 years) met the required physical activity levels (Nordstrøm et al. 2013:4395). Furthermore, individuals living with DS were the least active of these three groups. Another study reported that young children living with DS (3–10 years) did not meet the vigorous activity requirements per day when compared to their non-DS peers (Whitt-

Glover et al. 2006:158). Finally, a review article reiterated that children and adolescents living with DS did not meet the required amount of aerobic physical activity (Pitetti et al. 2013:47). Moreover, they indicated that the amount of physical activity decreased from childhood to adulthood. This may indicate that the root of a habitually sedentary lifestyle develops at a very young age (Boer 2015:31).

Nevertheless, it is recommended that future studies focus on practical strategies to motivate this population to be habitually active from a young age (Boer 2015:31; Kerstiens & Green 2015:192; Pitetti et al. 2013:47). In fact, Rubin et al. (1998:175) illustrated that it should be a major public health concern to identify opportunities for this population to be physically active and to achieve an optimal body composition. Wuang and Su (2012:841) reported that those children living with DS who had better cognitive and motor functions engaged in physical activities more often. The focus should perhaps be to target the individuals who do not possess these attributes. Additionally, individuals with a high BMI do not necessarily have to be targeted as Nordstrøm et al. (2013:4395) reported no association between physical activity levels and BMI in adolescents and adults living with DS. However, they did not distinguish between moderate and vigorous physical activity as in the study by Whitt-Glover et al. (2006:158). These authors stipulated that children living with DS should spend more time in vigorous physical activity that may prevent obesity and secure future health.

■ Ageing in adults living with Down syndrome

There has been a consistent trend toward an increased life expectancy in almost all developed and developing countries throughout the 20th century (Bittles et al. 2002:471). The investigators reported median life expectancies of 74.0, 67.6, and 58.6 years for people with mild, moderate and severe levels of intellectual disability. Carmeli et al. (2002:107) regard the evolution of medical technology and improvements in the quality of social and health care as major reasons for the increased life expectancy amongst people with ID. The number of people over the age of 60 years with lifelong developmental delays is predicted to double by 2030 (Barnhart & Connolly 2007:1400). This is also the case for DS individuals as 80% of this population lives past 30 years of age (Goodman & Miedaner 1998). In fact, life expectancy for DS individuals has been increasing from an average age of 9 years in 1929, to 12 years in 1949, 35 years in 1982 and currently to 55 years (Bittles & Glasson 2004:283). Torr et al. (2010:70) also found that the life expectancy of DS individuals increased vastly in the last three decades, which have led to an increased amount of DS adults living well into middle and old age.

Unfortunately, increasing age brings forth age-associated health problems. Carmeli et al. (2005:300) stated that increased life expectancy in the intellectually disabled population relates to an increase in the incidence of ageing disease and functional debility. Moreover, adults with ID tend to demonstrate premature signs of ageing, characterised by changes in body composition, functional decline and increased morbidity (Carfi et al. 2014:51; Carmeli et al. 2004; Oliver et al. 1998:1365; Terblanche & Boer 2013:834; Torr et al. 2010:70). In the DS population, the incidence of age-related diseases, such as Alzheimer's and diabetes, increases after the age of 30 or 35 (Folin et al. 2003:267; Krinsky-McHale et al. 2002:198). Shamas-Ud-Din (2002:167) stated that almost all DS individuals who progress beyond 40 years develop Alzheimer's disease. In combination with other health-related problems, these setbacks are further exacerbated as most individuals with DS live sedentary lifestyles (Esposito et al. 2012:109; Fernhall et al. 1996:366; Nordstrøm et al. 2013:4395; Shields et al. 2009:307). The ability to enjoy a mobile, active and independent lifestyle later in life depends largely on how well individuals maintain their functional fitness level, as most of the age-related physical decline is preventable and reversible through proper attention to daily physical needs (Rikli & Jones 2013).

■ Functional fitness and exercise in adults living with Down syndrome

The functional fitness of individuals living with DS is poor compared to the general population and to those living with ID but without DS (Baynard et al. 2004:1285, 2008:1984; Boer 2015:32; Eberhard, Eterradossi & Rapacchi 1989:167; Fernhall & Pitetti 2001:1657; Fernhall et al. 1996:366; Guerra, Pitetti & Fernhall 2003:1604; Pitetti & Fernhall 2004:219). The functional fitness of individuals living with DS may be poor because of the set of health, cognitive physiological, and psycho-social traits predisposing many of them to limited exercise (Boer 2015:32; Pitetti et al. 2013:47). Poor aerobic capacity is considered to be a risk factor for cardiovascular diseases and can result in reduced life expectancy for individuals living with DS (González-Agüero et al. 2010:720). Low levels of functional fitness may cause functional deterioration and reduce bone mineral density. This may aggravate existing clinical conditions (González-Agüero et al. 2010:717) and increase the risk of falls.

However, it has been reported that adults, adolescents and children living with DS can improve parameters associated with functional fitness (Boer & De Beer 2019:1453; Boer & Moss 2016a:322; Cowley et al. 2010:388, 2011:2229; Gupta, Rao & Sd 2011:425; Mendonca et al. 2013:353; Mendonca, Pereira & Fernhall 2011:37; Mendonca & Pereira 2009:33; Shields & Taylor 2010:187). Exercise strategies, such as aerobic training, resistance training, combined aerobic and resistance training, as well as interval training, have proven to be effective.

■ Assessing functional fitness in adults living with Down syndrome

If adults living with DS are able to improve their functional fitness (considering that they are mostly overweight, sedentary and suffer from many clinical conditions), how would one monitor their overall functional fitness?

Individuals in the general population (children, adults and elderly adults) and those living with physical and intellectual disabilities have measuring instruments to assess functional fitness (Boer 2015:33; Meredith & Welk 2010; Rikli & Jones 2013; Winnick & Short 2014). Functional fitness includes parameters such as flexibility, balance, aerobic capacity, functional capacity, and muscular strength and endurance (ch. 2). Unfortunately, adults living with DS do not have a standardised battery of instruments to measure functional fitness (Boer 2015:33). Currently, individuals living with DS are pooled with individuals living with ID without DS, even though the presence of DS negatively affects test performance (Baynard et al. 2004:1285, 2008:1984; Boer 2010:33; Pitetti & Fernhall 2004:219).

A standardised battery of test items is especially important in a population known to suffer from many health, functional and physical limitations. As such, research and academic scholars do not have a standardised set of functional norms with which to measure these individuals. Consequently, the academic scholar or exercise specialist cannot diagnose specific weaknesses and strengths or healthy and unhealthy zones of fitness. These unhealthy zones warn health practitioners when intervention is needed to pro-actively prevent future conditions or diseases. Furthermore, if a proper diagnosis of strengths and weaknesses cannot be made, training programs cannot be tailored to the specific needs of the individual. Moreover, the effect of a particular training program or intervention cannot be studied.

■ Rationale for developing the functional fitness test battery for adults with Down syndrome

In the section 'Ageing in adults living with Down syndrome', it was stated that the life expectancy of individuals living with DS is increasing. However, many individuals living with DS are also developing concomitant ageing diseases and conditions. As a result, individuals may lose their ability to function independently. In the past, health practitioners did not have access to standardised functional fitness tests for persons living with DS to assess their health and functional fitness. As such, practitioners had to use their own subjective knowledge for evaluation, assessment and exercise prescription. The functional fitness test battery (FFTB) was developed to improve the holistic assessment of functional fitness unique to the needs of adults living with DS. If functional fitness can be monitored early in life, and monitored over time, many physical and functional deficiencies could be prevented or reversed. In doing so, the quality of life will be improved for this susceptible group of individuals.

■ What are the uses of the functional fitness test battery for adults living with Down syndrome?

Adults living with DS can be assessed on various physical aspects such as balance, flexibility, muscular strength, functional fitness and aerobic capacity (ch. 4) to determine areas of strengths or weaknesses. An adult's test score can be compared to norm-referenced tables of other DS adults (ch. 3). The norm-referenced tables are categorised according to gender and age (every 15 years) providing a more specific breakdown of test performance compared to peers. The norm-referenced tables were obtained from 371 adults living with DS. This will provide the individual with an idea of how he or she fairs compared to other DS adults.

In addition to norm-referenced tables, criterion-referenced values are also provided. These standards are recommended minimum values needed for independent functioning later in life (ch. 3).

The FFTB for adults living with DS can also be used for research purposes. As the FFTB provides reliability and validity for all test items, it can be used to monitor improvements after an intervention period, longitudinal studies, or correlational and prediction studies.

Information from the FFTB can be used to prescribe exercise or other intervention strategies for adults living with DS. If an adult performs well on the aerobic test item but poorly on upper body strength, training could be tailored to the specific needs of the individual.

Additionally, an instrument of test items could act as motivation to improve or maintain fitness. Some adults might be competitive and would like to compete with those on higher percentiles, whereas others would like to improve as to meet the minimum required standards.

Lastly, this book could provide the necessary information for the managerial staff working at intellectually disabled care centres. Most of the senior managers at these centres are ill-equipped to understand the importance of adequate functional fitness for adults living with DS. With the help of a research scholar or exercise specialist and the contents of this book, managerial staff will be equipped to initiate the process of functional fitness assessment at respective care centres for adults living with DS.

■ Why is the functional fitness test battery for adults living with Down syndrome so easy to perform?

Firstly, the FFTB is holistic and comprehensive. It covers all facets of functional fitness. Many other instruments focus on one facet such as balance, flexibility or lower body strength. The FFTB covers all physiological parameters to assess functional fitness (ch. 2 and ch. 4).

The tests presented herein are field based. None of the tests require laboratory-based tests. Consequently, the tests can easily be performed at a care centre for people living with IDs. Minimal space requirements are needed except for the two aerobic test items (20 m by 10 m). Additionally, limited equipment is required in order to assess the field tests (app. C). Moreover, any research scholar in the field of exercise science or adapted physical activity with adequate knowledge of the testing methods or procedures (ch. 4) and experience in working with DS individuals will be able to administer the tests.

The FFTB provides norm- and criterion-referenced tables that the adults living with DS can use for personal comparison and assessment. This is an uncomplicated task (ch. 3). The tables of the FFTB are structured in such a way that one can monitor one's own test performance in relation to adults of the same gender and age category.

A summarised appendix is attached with the key points for using the FFTB (app. H).

■ Who is this test battery designed for and who can administer the tests?

All adults living with DS (18 years and older) may perform the tests associated with this book. However, it is advised that those with mosaic type DS (1% of all DS individuals) do not compare their scores with the norm-referenced tables as their functional fitness abilities are much higher than their peers without the mosaic type DS. It is important to note, as stated previously, that adults living with DS should be cleared to perform the activities presented in this book by their primary physician by completing the adapted physical activity readiness questionnaire (app. G). The reason for this is that many individuals living with DS suffer from congenital heart diseases or muscular-skeletal problems which is contraindicative to exercise.

Adults living with DS are presented with different levels of intelligence. These tests were standardised on those individuals who are capable of understanding test instructions and procedures. Adults with severe ID may not be able to perform some of the tests presented in this book. The individual administering the tests should have the ability to demonstrate and explain clearly and meticulously to adults living with DS. The person should have experience in working with individuals living with DS. Most individuals living with DS have to be constantly motivated during the tests with phrases such as 'you can do this', 'keep working' and similar phrases. If constant motivation during tests are not provided, the individuals will not present their best effort. In most cases, individuals need to be motivated to go faster, harder or better as their motivational levels may be insufficient. Consequently, the person administering the tests needs experience in working with individuals living with DS and adequate knowledge of tests involving balance, flexibility, strength, functional and aerobic activities. Therefore, an academic or research scholar with experience in the field of adapted physical activity would be the most suitable candidate to assess functional fitness.

■ Summary

Functional fitness is defined as having the physical capacity to perform normal everyday activities safely and independently without undue fatigue. It has been reported that adults living with DS suffer from many conditions and have low functional fitness. Adults living with DS do not have a unique, holistic and standardised instrument to assess functional fitness. They are often pooled with individuals living with ID (without DS) even though they have marked differences in functional fitness. Many adults living with DS cannot perform the tests developed for individuals living with ID. There was a need to develop a standardised battery of test items specifically for adults living with DS.

The FFTB is easy to perform, field based and requires minimal equipment. Any academic or research scholar or exercise specialist in adapted physical activity with experience in working with adults living with DS can administer the tests. The participant's health practitioner should be consulted before testing using the adapted physical activity readiness questionnaire (app. G). All information pertaining to testing procedures (ch. 4), order of tests (app. D), equipment and space needed (app. C), participant score sheet (app. E and app. F), and norm- and criterion-referenced tables (ch. 3) are provided in this book.

Conceptual framework: The functional fitness battery of test items

■ Functional fitness versus physical fitness

Many adapted physical activity research scholar and academia have opted to use the term 'functional fitness' as opposed to 'physical fitness' in non-athletic populations to incorporate terms such as health and functional capacity (Boer 2010:17; Brill 2004:5; Rikli & Jones 2013). This is usually the case for elderly and disabled populations but also in populations with chronic medical conditions. It could be argued that these special populations need a certain measure of fitness that would enhance health and functional abilities, but which is not similar to the high levels of physical fitness expected of athletic populations (Boer 2010:17).

It has been established that various physical parameters are directly associated with functional capacity (Brill 2004:5; Cowley et al. 2010:388; Morey et al. 1998:715; Rikli & Jones 2013:12; Singh et al. 2006:4). Rikli and Jones (2013:12) as well as Brill (2004:5) stated that it is imperative to study the extent to which various components of physical fitness contribute to functionality. The ability to perform common tasks such as shopping, household chores, gardening and recreational activities requires the ability to

How to cite: Boer, P.-H., 2021, 'Conceptual framework: The functional fitness battery of test items', in *Functional fitness for adults living with Down syndrome*, pp. 15–22, AOSIS, Cape Town. https://doi.org/10.4102/aosis.2021. BK252.02

perform various functions including walking, stair climbing, carrying, twisting, turning, pushing and pulling (Boer 2010:17). In turn, these functions require physical characteristics such as muscular strength, aerobic endurance, flexibility and balance. The 'Procedural elements related to test selection' section will discuss how these physical parameters were selected for the FFTB for adults living with DS.

■ Procedural elements related to test selection

When we started the development of the FFTB for adults with DS in 2009, various standardised tests were available for individuals with ID (Boer 2015:3). The standardised tests and manuals available for youngsters with ID included: The Brockport Physical Test (BPFT) (Winnick & Short 2014) (previous edition, 1999), The Special Fitness Test (American Alliance for Health, Physical Education and Recreation 1976), The Motor Fitness Test Manual for the Moderately Mentally Retarded (Johnson & Londeree 1976); The FAIT Physical Fitness Test for Mildly and Moderately Mentally Retarded Students (Fait & Dunn 1984); The Project Active level II (Vodola 1978); Ohio State SIGMA (Loovis & Ersing 1979); and The Youth Fitness Test for mildly mentally retarded (American Alliance for Health, Physical Education, Recreation and Dance 1978). Most of these studies concentrated on ages of up to 18 years with one fitness battery extending to 20 years (Boer 2015:3). None of these studies focused explicitly on a population of (1) DS individuals and (2) ID or DS adults (Boer 2010:33). Moreover, all these batteries include ID as a whole with no studies establishing certain recommendations with reference to exercise tests for DS individuals. In fact, Winnick and Short (2014) acknowledge that the BPFT makes no distinction between those with and without DS despite evidence that the presence of DS negatively affects fitness test performance. As such, there is no descriptive information on the physical and functional tests available in an exclusive DS population. This information is however vital, as there is clear evidence that DS adults have marked reductions in physical and functional capabilities compared to those with ID, but without DS (Baynard et al. 2004:1285, 2008:1984; Boer 2010:33, 2015:32; Eberhard et al. 1989:167; Fernhall & Pitetti 2001:1657; Fernhall et al. 1996:366; Guerra et al. 2003:1604; Pitetti & Fernhall 2004:219).

In an extensive literature review, all available instruments to assess functional fitness were identified. All final functional fitness tests went through a very carefully selected and rigorous process (Boer & Moss 2016b:179). The same selection process was also followed by Winnick and Short (2014); Rikli and Jones (2013); Hilgenkamp, Van Wijck and Evenhuis (2013:34); Hilgenkamp, Van Wijck and Evenhuis (2012:158); and Hilgenkamp, Van Wijck and Evenhuis (2010:1030). Using the information provided by the BPFT (Winnick & Short 2014); the Senior Fitness Test (SFT) (Rikli & Jones 2013); Hilgenkamp et al. (2012:158) and the ACSM (2013), six parameters to describe functional fitness (balance, flexibility, functional ability, muscular strength and endurance, cardiovascular endurance, BMI) were selected (Boer & Moss 2016b:179). A thorough literature study was conducted to identify all possible measuring instruments based on their existing functionality, reliability and validity (ch. 3). A 3-month pilot study ensued, after which the test choices were further refined with the help of research scholars in the field of adapted physical education, DS research and disability sport. Feasibility analyses were also performed and conducted at three intellectually disabled care centres in the Western Cape of South Africa. Feasibility encompassed several aspects, amongst others: demands of the test to participants, level of difficulty of the instructions to the participant, level of difficulty of the execution of the task itself, duration of tests and completion rates of the test. Final test items were selected from the Bruininks–Oseretsky Test of Motor Proficiency (BOTMP), the BPFT and the SFT. The 'Overview of the importance of adequate aerobic capacity, musculoskeletal functional balance and an optimal body mass index' section provides a brief overview of the importance of adequate aerobic capacity, musculoskeletal functional balance and optimal BMI. The final instrument contained two balance test items, two flexibility items, five muscular strength and endurance items, two aerobic items, one functional task and the parameter BMI.

After test selection, the feasibility of these tests was determined and reported to be excellent as shown in 371 adults living with DS (Terblanche & Boer 2013:826). All test items showed good reliability with intraclass correlation coefficients (ICCs) of 0.9 or higher (Boer & Moss 2016b:176). The discriminant validity has also been reported for all the test items in adults living with DS (Terblanche & Boer 2013:826). The logical or criterion-related validity is also described and reported (Boer & Moss 2016c:2575; Rikli & Jones 2013:24; Winnick & Short 2014:29). Detailed information regarding the feasibility, reliability and validity of these test items are described in Chapter 3.

■ Overview of the importance of adequate aerobic capacity, musculoskeletal functional balance and an optimal body mass index

Aerobic endurance

Aerobic activities refer to the ability of the large muscle groups to function for an extended period of time because of the capacity of the cardiopulmonary system which provides oxygenated blood to the muscles (Winnick & Short 2014:7). Walking long distances or participating in recreational activities such as swimming, cycling, tennis or bowls requires an adequate aerobic capacity. The aerobic capacity of non-disabled and disabled individuals decreases over time and it is important to maintain an adequate aerobic capacity or to control the rate of decline (Rikli & Jones 2013:14; Terblanche & Boer 2013:826;

Winnick & Short 2014:7). Maintaining an adequate level of aerobic capacity is important for functional ability and cardiovascular health. A poor aerobic capacity has been correlated with clinical conditions such as cardiovascular disease, hypertension, obesity and diabetes (González-Agüero et al. 2010:717; Winnick & Short 2014:7).

Musculoskeletal functioning

Musculoskeletal functioning comprises of three facets (muscular strength, muscular endurance and flexibility). The relationship between musculoskeletal functioning and functional fitness has a logical basis and can have far-reaching consequences later in life (Winnick & Short 2014:7).

Firstly, muscular strength includes activities where objects such as a bag of groceries need to be lifted or when an object needs to be pushed or pulled (upper body strength) or climbing out of the bath (lower body strength). Secondly, muscular endurance is required for activities that necessitate repeated muscle contractions such as mowing the lawn, carrying a grocery bag, climbing stairs, maintaining posture or performing a recreational activity such as tennis or bowls. Thirdly, flexibility is required for reaching, bending, lifting, changing clothes or driving. Maintaining lower body flexibility could also prevent lower back pain and musculoskeletal injuries. The flexibility of adults living with DS is good and should not be overtrained (Boer 2010). All three of these facets can be improved with structured training in adults living with DS. It has been reported that the musculoskeletal functioning of adults living with DS decreases as they age and the maintenance thereof remains essential (Terblanche & Boer 2013:826).

Balance

Adequate balance is an important facet for individuals living with DS. Good static and dynamic balance could prevent falls and improve walking economy. Everyday living activities such as walking and turning, showering, hiking on uneven terrain and recreational activities such as tennis and golf need proper static or dynamic balance. Postural control in children and adolescents with DS has been shown to be poor compared to general population (Cabeza-Ruiz et al. 2011:23; Galli et al. 2008:1274; Rigoldi et al. 2011:170). Moreover, abnormalities in the functioning of the vestibular apparatus of individuals with DS and challenges experienced by these individuals in extracting relevant information have been reported by Cabeza-Ruiz et al. (2011:23). Villarroya et al. (2012:1294) reported that an appropriate rehabilitation program consisting of somatosensory stimuli could be a useful measure to improve balance for adolescents with DS. The static and dynamic balance of adults living with DS decreases as they age and should be maintained over time (Terblanche & Boer 2013:835).

Body mass index

As reported in Chapter 1, many adults living with DS are overweight or obese. Obesity or a high BMI can have a marked influence on a person's functional fitness. A higher BMI has also been reported to have a negative correlation with aerobic capacity in adults living with DS (Salaun & Berthouze-Aranda 2012:231). The individuals with the lowest BMI have the highest aerobic capacity. Additionally, individuals with higher BMIs have serious difficulty performing activities such as climbing stairs and walking long distances to the same extent as those with optimal body weight (Rikli & Jones 2013:13). It has been recommended that BMI is included as a functional fitness parameter in the FFTB as overweight individuals are more likely to be disabled in later years (Bertapelli et al. 2016:181; Wong et al. 2015:139).

■ Functional fitness parameters for the functional fitness test battery for adults living with Down syndrome

The importance of various physical parameters for functional fitness has been described. The FFTB for adults living with DS was constructed based on the evidence and information provided by Winnick and Short (2014:29), Rikli and Jones (2013:23), and Hilgenkamp et al. (2012:158). The FFTB consists of various physical items to assess functional fitness for adults living with DS. Fourteen test items were included in the FFTB. Two test items were selected from the BOTMP; five test items from the BPFT and seven test items from the SFT. The test items include the measurement of height and weight to determine BMI and comprise of two aerobic items, two balance items, two flexibility items, one functional item, and five muscular strength and endurance items (Box 2.1).

Box 2.1: A brief overview of the functional fitness parameters for the functional fitness test battery for adults living with Down syndrome.

Aerobic endurance	
Test item 1	**6-minute walk distance test (SFT)**
Purpose	To assess the aerobic capacity which involves brisk walking which is important for walking longer distances or climbing stairs.
Description	Number of metres that can be walked around a 50-yard (45 m and 72 m) rectangular course.
Test item 2	**16-metre PACER test (BPFT)**
Purpose	To assess the aerobic capacity which involves running.
Description	Number of shuttles (16 m) that can be run on an audio signal (tempo/pace increases with time).

Box 2.1 continues on the next page→

Box 2.1 (Continues...): A brief overview of the functional fitness parameters for the functional fitness test battery for adults living with Down syndrome.

Musculoskeletal functioning: Flexibility	
Test item 3	**Chair sit-and-reach test (SFT)**
Purpose	To assess lower body flexibility which is important for correct posture and activities such as bending or reaching.
Description	In a seated position, the participant stretches as far forward as possible with one leg extended and fingers reaching towards the toes.
Test item 4	**Back scratch test (SFT)**
Purpose	To assess lower body flexibility which is important for correct posture and activities such as bending or reaching.
Description	In a seated position, the participant stretches as far forward as possible with one leg extended and fingers reaching towards the toes.
Musculoskeletal functioning: Muscular strength	
Test item 5	**Handgrip strength (BPFT)**
Purpose	To assess forearm strength needed to lift objects or opening a jar.
Description	The participant squeezes the hand-held dynamometer with as much force as possible.
Musculoskeletal functioning: Muscular endurance	
Test item 6	**Isometric push-up (BPFT)**
Purpose	To assess upper body endurance needed for pushing or pulling objects (vacuum machine or lawn mower).
Description	Participant assumes the push-up position and holds the position for as long as possible.
Test item 7	**Trunk lift (BPFT)**
Purpose	To assess trunk strength which is important for posture whilst sitting and standing.
Description	From a prone position, the participant lifts his trunk to a maximum position.
Test item 8	**Modified curl-up (BPFT)**
Purpose	To assess abdominal strength and endurance needed for many activities such as raising from a prone position or when twisting or turning movements are involved.
Description	From a prone position, the participant curls up slowly by sliding the fingers from the thighs to the knee.
Test item 9	**30-second chair stand test (SFT)**
Purpose	To assess lower body strength and endurance needed for activities such as climbing stairs, walking and getting out of a car.
Description	Number of full stands from a seated position performed within 30 s is recorded.

Box 2.1 continues on the next page→

Box 2.1 (Continues...): A brief overview of the functional fitness parameters for the functional fitness test battery for adults living with Down syndrome.

Balance: Static balance	
Test item 10	**Standing on one leg (stalk stand) (BOTMP)**
Purpose	Assessing static balance which is important for extended periods of standing and the prevention of falls.
Description	The participant stands on one leg, with the other leg bent at 90°, and the hands on the hips.
Balance: Dynamic balance	
Test item 11	**Walking on a balance beam (BOTMP)**
Purpose	To assess dynamic balance which is important for balance whilst mobile (walking on the pavement and hiking trails).
Description	Participant walks on a 3.05-m balance beam (10.16 cm wide) and attempts to walk a maximum of six steps.
Balance: Functional ability	
Test item 12	**8-foot up-and-go test (SFT)**
Purpose	To assess the functional ability of the participant that mimics a task of everyday living such as getting up from a chair.
Description	Number of seconds required to get up from a seated position, walk eight feet (2.44 m), turn and return to a seated position is recorded.
Test item 13 and 14	**Body mass and height: Body mass index (SFT)**
Purpose	To calculate one's ratio of body weight relative to height because of the importance of optimal weight for functional mobility.
Description	The participant's height and weight is taken and substituted into a formula to calculate BMI.

Note: SFT, Senior Fitness Test; BPFT, Brockport Physical Fitness Test; BOTMP, Bruininks–Oseretsky Test of Motor Proficiency. Detailed test descriptions are provided in Chapter 4 and in Appendix D.

■ Summary

The FFTB was developed to evaluate, monitor and improve the functional fitness of adults living with DS. Five components were identified and deemed necessary for monitoring functional fitness:

1. aerobic capacity
2. musculoskeletal functioning, including muscular strength, endurance and flexibility
3. balance
4. functional ability
5. BMI.

The FFTB uses test items that are:

1. adapted to adults living with DS
2. reliable and valid
3. used to assess a variety of performance levels
4. easy to administer with minimal equipment requirements
5. sensitive to detect changes.

Tests were selected from the BOTMP, the BPFT and the SFT.

Test feasibility, reliability, validity and percentile norms

◼ Standardised fitness tests

Standardised fitness tests must demonstrate adequate feasibility, reliability and validity. The feasibility, reliability and validity should be reported in the population being tested. A feasible test is one where most of the participants can complete a specific test successfully and obtain a test score. A reliable test is one that can consistently and repeatedly measure the same test score for a specific individual. Consequently, the test should be free from measurement error. Validity is important as the test should measure what it is purported to measure. In other words, the test should correlate well with a criterion or a gold standard-test. In some cases, a criterion is not available and validity is based on logical or discriminant validity.

Once the feasibility, reliability and validity of tests have been determined, performance scales can be developed in large epidemiological studies. This will enable test examiners to interpret test scores. If norm profile scales are used, the participant's score can be compared to peers of his or her age. Strengths and weaknesses in specific domains of functional fitness can then be identified and fitness programs can be tailored accordingly. However, criterion-referenced standards are better equipped to indicate the level of performance required in order to achieve a specific criterion such as being

How to cite: Boer, P.-H., 2021, 'Test feasibility, reliability, validity and percentile norms', in *Functional fitness for adults living with Down syndrome*, pp. 23–45, AOSIS, Cape Town. https://doi.org/10.4102/aosis.2021.BK252.03

healthy or independent. Norm- and criterion-referenced scales are discussed in greater detail in the latter part of this chapter.

■ Feasibility of the functional fitness test battery for adults living with Down syndrome

When the pilot study was performed for the identification and selection of test items, it was realised that many participants were not able to successfully complete a number of the initial test items. These test items already included items adapted to the needs of the elderly or those living with ID without DS. As a result, feasibility had to be established to assess the percentage of participants who were able to successfully complete each particular test item. Consequently, the feasibility of all the selected tests had to be determined. The procedure of test selection and refinement is well-described in Chapter 2.

In a previous study, the feasibility of the functional fitness items in 371 adults living with DS was described (Terblanche & Boer 2013:826). The majority of tests revealed a 100% completion rate whereas three tests demonstrated close to 98% completion. A small number of participants were not able to complete the sit-and-reach test, isometric push-up and the 30-second chair stand test.

■ Reliability of the functional fitness test battery for adults living with Down syndrome

A reliable test is important as test-to-test variation should be minimal. Consistency of measurements should be optimal even when a test is performed 7 to 10 days apart. A reliable test score is also free from measurement error. The test-retest reliability of all functional fitness test items is reported in Table 3.1. Reliability of a test is best determined by a one-way analysis of variance (ANOVA) to determine the ICC between test and retest. The one-way ANOVA model treats all sources of measurement variation, including changes from day-to-day variation, as error. Results indicated that the ICC for all test items ranged from 0.90 to 0.98 (Table 3.1). Confidence intervals (95%) are also demonstrated in this table. Standard error of measurement (SEM) scores and minimal detectable change (MDC) scores at 90% confidence interval also indicated acceptable precision (SEM < SD/2) and low variability (Table 3.1). Previous studies have also determined the test-retest reliability for elderly individuals in the general population (SFT [Rikli & Jones 2013:35]), adolescents living with ID (BPFT [Winnick & Short 2014:29]) and elderly individuals living with ID (Hilgenkamp, Van Wijck & Evenhuis 2012:158).

TABLE 3.1: Test-retest reliability of 12 functional test items in adult persons with Down syndrome.

Test	Mean ± SD		ICC (95% CI)	SEM	MDC$_{90}$
	Test 1	Test 2			
SOOL left (s)	5.9 (3.7)	6.0 (3.6)	0.98 (0.96–0.99)	0.53	1.23
SOOL right (s)	5.5 (3.5)	5.9 (3.6)	0.93 (0.88–0.96)	0.92	2.14
WOBB (steps)	4.3 (2.1)	4.6 (2.1)	0.93 (0.88–0.96)	0.55	1.28
Back scratch left (cm)	−4.2 (10.1)	−4.1 (9.8)	0.99 (0.97–0.99)	1.24	2.89
Back scratch right (cm)	−2.3 (8.6)	−2.6 (8.2)	0.98 (0.97–0.99)	1.15	2.68
S&R left (cm)	8.2 (8.8)	8.9 (9.1)	0.98 (0.97–0.99)	1.21	2.83
S&R right (cm)	8.4 (8.7)	8.9 (9.1)	0.98 (0.97–0.99)	1.09	2.55
Chair stand (n)	14.4 (1.9)	14.4 (2.1)	0.94 (0.89–0.97)	0.48	1.12
Isometric push-up (s)	42.8 (38.8)	44.2 (37.0)	0.99 (0.97–0.99)	4.75	11.08
Handgrip strength (kg)	26.3 (8.2)	26.5 (8.1)	0.98 (0.95–0.99)	1.29	3.02
Modified curl-up (n)	37.8 (26.5)	39.3 (26.9)	0.99 (0.98–0.99)	2.65	6.15
Trunk lift (cm)	27.8 (9.3)	27.9 (10.5)	0.96 (0.93–0.98)	1.91	4.47
8-foot up-and-go (s)	5.5 (1.2)	5.4 (1.1)	0.94 (0.89–0.97)	0.30	0.70
16-metre PACER (n)	22.8 (13.5)	23.0 (13.8)	0.99 (0.98–0.99)	1.54	3.60
6-minute walk distance (m)	518.4 (81.5)	513.1 (82.3)	0.93 (0.88–0.96)	21.24	49.57

Source: Boer and Moss (2016b:n.p.).

Note: Data are presented as mean and SD. Intraclass correlation coefficient and 95% CIs are shown, as well as SEM and MDC$_{90}$. SOOL, standing on one leg; S&R, chair sit-and-reach test; WOBB, walking on balance beam.

Reliability for the same test items in different populations

Rikli and Jones (2013:35) demonstrated ICC values similar to the results depicted in Table 3.1 for the 30-second chair stand test ($R = 0.89$), 6-minute walk distance test ($R = 0.94$), chair sit-and-reach ($R = 0.95$), back scratch ($R = 0.96$) and the 8-foot up-and-go test ($R = 0.95$) in elderly individuals in the general population.

Winnick and Short (1998:20) reported test-retest ICC values ranging from 0.82 to 0.98 in adolescents living with ID measured 2 weeks apart for the back scratch test, modified curl-up test, trunk lift test, 16-metre PACER test and isometric push-up test.

Hilgenkamp et al. (2012:160) performed test-retest reliability in older adults living with ID and found ICC values (same day interval and 2-week interval) for the 30-second chair stand test ($R = 0.72$; $R = 0.65$) and handgrip strength ($R = 0.94$; $R = 0.90$).

Wuang and Su (2009:847) determined the test-retest reliability ($R = 0.99$) of the balance tests (standing on one leg and walking on the balance beam) in adolescents living with ID.

Regarding the 6-minute walk distance test, an ICC value of $R = 0.98$ was demonstrated in adults living with ID (Nasuti, Stuart-Hill & Temple 2013:31) and no significant difference was found between test and retest for adolescents living with DS (Casey, Wang & Osterling 2012:2068). The ICC score (R = 0.96) for the 6-minute walk distance test was also shown to be very high for adults and elderly adults living with ID (Guerra-Balic et al. 2015:144).

■ Validity

When tests are administered to participants, they should capture what they are purported to measure. For example, it should be shown that the 30-second chair stand test actually measures leg strength. Therefore, the 30-second chair stand test should be compared with a test that has already been demonstrated to indicate leg strength (criterion-related validity). Tests can also demonstrate other sources of validity when assessed after a training program or between different groups (discriminant validity). Criterion, content (logical) or discriminant validity is discussed briefly in this section.

▨ Criterion-related validity

Criterion-related validity is calculated as the extent to which one test correlates to an existing criterion which has already been shown to be valid. It is best to assess the criterion validity of an existing test with the gold standard of that construct. Pearson correlation coefficients or regression analysis is often used to assess validity.

▨ Content-related validity

Content-related or logical validity can be described as the extent to which a certain performance test reflects a specific domain of content such as functional fitness. Detailed literature review studies are often employed to determine logical validity in addition to subjective decisions by expert academic scholars in the appropriate field of study. Content-related validity for all functional fitness tests is described in detail in Chapter 2. The selection of appropriate tests for adults living with DS followed a rigorous and thorough literature review of the construct functional fitness. This was followed by the evaluation of test items with established reliability and validity in other functionally limited populations with the assistance of experts in the field of adapted physical activity and actively involved in exercise or functional testing of DS individuals. Discriminant validity refers to situations where a specific test is able to discriminate between participants (active versus inactive, pre-training versus post-training or between different age groups).

■ Validity of the functional fitness test battery for adults living with Down syndrome

Discriminant validity has been determined for all test items in a large epidemiological study with 371 adults living with DS (Terblanche & Boer 2013:826). All functional fitness tests were able to discriminate between adults living with DS in different age groups (18–25; 26–35; 36–45; > 45) except for lower body flexibility and handgrip strength (Table 3.2). However, Cowley et al. (2010:388) demonstrated that the timed up-and-go test (similar to the 8-foot up-and-go test) discriminates well between those with high or low aerobic capacity and leg strength in adults living with DS.

TABLE 3.2: Discriminant validity in adults living with Down syndrome.

Test items	Participants	Age categories				
		Combined	18–25	26–35	36–45	> 45
BMI	Men	29.9 (5.6)	30.8 (6.0)	30.1 (6.0)	28.9 (5.0)	28.2 (4.5)
	Women	31.9 (6.4)	32.0 (6.2)	31.4 (6.7)	33.1 (6.4)	31.1 (5.9)
Standing on one leg *	Men	6.2 (3.6)	7.0 (3.5)	6.6 (3.6)	5.8 (3.5)	4.4 (3.4)
	Women	4.8 (3.6)	5.6 (3.7)	5.5 (3.8)	4.2 (3.3)	3.0 (3.0)
Walking on balance beam *	Men	3.6 (2.3)	4.1 (2.7)	4.1 (2.2)	3.1 (2.7)	2.5 (2.2)
	Women	3.0 (2.5)	4.0 (2.3)	3.6 (2.5)	1.8 (1.3)	1.4 (2.3)
Back scratch (cm) *	Men	−4.3 (10.8)	−2.5 (11.2)	−5.4 (11.8)	−3.9 (10.1)	−6.0 (9.2)
	Women	−6.1 (9.4)	−2.6 (8.9)	−5.8 (9.5)	−8.9 (9.7)	−7.5 (8.1)
Chair sit-and-reach (cm)	Men	6.2 (10.0)	7.5 (11.2)	7.9 (9.9)	5.0 (9.6)	3.4 (7.9)
	Women	6.7 (9.1)	8.3 (10.9)	6.8 (8.7)	5.3 (8.8)	5.9 (6.4)
Chair stands (cm) *	Men	12.2 (2.5)	13.2 (2.4)	12.7 (2.4)	11.8 (2.5)	10.7 (2.3)
	Women	12.3 (2.6)	12.5 (2.6)	12.8 (2.5)	12.2 (2.5)	11.0 (2.9)
Isometric push-up *	Men	50.7 (38.9)	55.8 (38.8)	54.3 (47.3)	51.2 (31.6)	33.9 (30.5)
	Women	29.7 (25.2)	31.3 (26.8)	36.3 (26.0)	26.2 (21.1)	20.1 (24.6)
Handgrip strength (kg)	Men	29.8 (8.5)	30.1 (8.1)	30.6 (9.3)	29.3 (8.2)	29.0 (8.0)
	Women	20.7 (5.5)	20.7 (4.8)	21.8 (5.5)	20.9 (5.6)	18.4 (6.2)
Modified curl-up *	Men	22.4 (27.2)	28.3 (30.1)	21.9 (27.5)	22.3 (26.4)	13.0 (20.6)
	Women	13.5 (21.9)	14.0 (24.1)	20.0 (26.4)	10.0 (13.1)	6.6 (17.8)
Trunk lift (cm) *	Men	29.3 (8.9)	29.6 (8.4)	31.8 (9.2)	29.9 (8.1)	22.8 (8.1)
	Women	26.3 (7.5)	29.1 (7.4)	28.4 (6.3)	24.0 (6.9)	21.4 (7.2)
8-foot up-and-go (s) *	Men	6.2 (1.5)	5.8 (1.2)	6.2 (1.5)	6.3 (1.5)	7.1 (1.7)
	Women	6.7 (1.9)	6.1 (1.2)	6.1 (1.1)	6.9 (1.5)	8.4 (3.0)
16-metre PACER (n) *	Men	21.1 (15.1)	25.4 (14.9)	23.6 (17.5)	19.5 (13.2)	11.8 (8.7)
	Women	12.2 (9.5)	14.1 (7.7)	15.4 (12.1)	10.4 (7.7)	6.3 (5.3)

Source: Terblanche and Boer (2013:n.p.).

Note: BMI, Body Mass Index; *, Significantly different amelioration between age groups.

Discriminant validity has also been reported with significant improvements in the 6-minute walk distance test, 16-metre PACER test, modified curl-up test, 8-foot up-and-go test, handgrip strength test and 30-second chair stand test after a training intervention in adults living with DS (Boer & De Beer 2019:1459; Boer & Moss 2016a:322; Carmeli et al. 2002:106; Chen, Ringenbach & Snow 2014:288).

Regarding criterion-related validity, the 6-minute walk distance test (R^2 = 0.75) and 16-metre PACER (R^2 = 0.86) tests have shown to be related (Boer & Moss 2016c:2575) to the gold standard VO_2 max (Fernhall et al. 1990:1065) (Tables 3.3 and 3.4). These results were shown specifically for adults with DS.

Content-related or logical validity for all functional fitness tests was described in detail in Chapter 2.

The 'Validity of the functional fitness test items in the general elderly or intellectually disabled populations' section will describe the validity of all functional fitness items as determined in the general elderly population and individuals living with ID.

TABLE 3.3: Predictors of peak VO_2 using demographic variables and the 16-metre PACER test as independent variables.

Predictive variable	Unstandardised (ß)	SE	t-value	p-value	Standardised estimate (ß)
Intercept	48.43	5.03	9.2	<0.01	/
16-metre PACER (n)	0.32	0.05	6.9	<0.01	0.59
BMI (kg/m²)	−0.45	0.13	−3.5	<0.01	−0.29
Gender	−2.88	0.96	−3.0	<0.01	−0.19
Age (yrs)	−0.13	0.05	−2.5	0.02	−0.15
R^2		0.86	Adjusted R^2		0.85

Source: Boer and Moss (2016c).
Note: VO_2 peak = 48.23 + 0.32 (16-metre PACER) − 0.45 (BMI) − 2.88 (Gender) − 0.13 (Age); Gender (1 male, 2 female).

TABLE 3.4: Predictors of peak VO_2 using demographic variables and the 6-minute walk distance test as independent variables.

Predictive variable	Unstandardised (ß)	SE	t-value	p-value	Standardised estimate (ß)
Intercept	30.27	8.03	3.8	<0.01	/
6MWD (m)	0.05	0.01	5.4	<0.01	0.53
BMI (kg/m²)	−0.70	0.15	−4.67	<0.01	−0.45
R^2	−	0.75	Adjusted R^2	−	0.74

Source: Boer and Moss (2016c).
BMI, body mass index; 6MWD, *6-minute walk distance*.

■ Validity of the functional fitness test items in the general elderly or intellectually disabled populations

This section presents a brief discussion of the background and validity evidence of the various functional fitness tests.

▨ Flexibility

☐ Chair sit-and-reach test

The chair sit-and-reach test was adapted from earlier versions of the floor sit-and-reach test (YMCA test battery & Fitnessgram) (Rikli & Jones 2013:18). Many adults living with DS suffer from obesity, muscle hypotonicity and low muscle strength. Therefore, the chair sit-and-reach test is more suitable as it is easier to perform than the original version. Our intensive pilot study demonstrated improved feasibility with this test to assess lower body flexibility.

Criterion-related validity for the chair sit-and-reach test has been demonstrated with goniometer-measured hamstring flexibility in elderly adults (Rikli & Jones 1998). Jones et al. (1998:338) reported that the chair sit-and-reach test was better correlated with goniometer-measured hamstring flexibility compared to the floor sit-and-reach test.

☐ Back scratch test

The back scratch test is a modified version of the Apley test. In the Apley test, participants also reached with one hand over the shoulder and the other behind the back but had to touch anatomical landmarks. The back scratch test is easier and more quantifiable in a field setting (Rikli & Jones 2013:18).

Only logical or content-related validity for this test has been reported by experts in the field (Woodward & Best 2000), as this test involves placing one hand behind the head and over the shoulder (shoulder flexion, external rotation and adduction) whereas stretching the hand behind the back involves shoulder extension, internal rotation and adduction. Reduced shoulder flexibility is associated with an increased chance of injury in later years (Chakravarty & Webley 1993:1359; Bassey et al. 1989:249). No single criterion exists for the Apley or back scratch test (Rikli & Jones 2013:16). Similar versions of this test are also found in other fitness batteries such as the Fitnessgram (Meredith & Welk 2010) and the BPFT (Winnick & Short 2014). Discriminant validity for this test has been reported in elderly individuals (Rikli 2000:89; Rikli & Jones 1999:162).

☐ Balance

Static balance is assessed with the stalk stand (standing on one leg). Construct validity has been determined by Lin et al. (2004:1343) in elderly individuals. Vellas et al. (1997:735) reported that the one-legged stand demonstrates discriminant validity as performance in this test is able to predict injurious falls. Dynamic balance was assessed when participants had to walk on a 3.05-m-long balance beam placed on the floor. Discriminant validity for dynamic balance has been reported by Carmeli et al. (2002:106) as dynamic balance can be improved after an intervention period.

▨ Muscular strength and endurance

☐ Leg strength

Rikli and Jones (2013:15) reported that this test was adapted from one that required participants to perform a certain number of stands in the quickest time possible. However, in this test, many participants could not obtain test scores as the test is time-based rather than count-based. With the 30-second chair stand test, everybody can obtain a test score even if it is one stand in the allocated 30 s. Jones et al. (1999:113) and Bohannon (1998:434) demonstrated adequate criterion-related validity with a maximum weight-adjusted leg press performance test and leg extension strength in elderly participants.

☐ Handgrip strength

Construct validity has been demonstrated with various functional tasks in the general elderly population (Abizanda et al. 2012:21). Handgrip strength is also used in other fitness batteries such as the BPFT (Winnick & Short 2014) and the Fitnessgram (Meredith & Welk 2010).

▨ Abdominal strength and upper body strength

The modified curl-up, isometric push-up and trunk lift have been shown to present logical validity in individuals living with ID (Winnick & Short 2014:29).

☐ Functional test

☐ 8-foot up-and-go test

This test is a modified version of the timed up-and-go test and has been correlated to various ADL (criterion-related validity) (Podsiadlo & Richardson 1991:142). These researchers and Rikli and Jones (1999:113) also reported discriminant validity for this test in elderly adults. The test has also been shown to discriminate well with an increased risk of falling if the test score is more than 8.5 s.

☐ Aerobic tests

☐ 6-minute walk distance test

The 6-minute walk distance test has also proved to be related to standardised treadmill protocols in the elderly population (Rikli & Jones 1998). The criterion-related validity for adolescents (r = 0.69) and adults (R^2 = 0.67) living with ID have also been determined for the 6-minute walk distance test (Elmahgoub et al. 2012:846; Nasuti et al. 2013:31).

☐ 16-metre PACER test

Fernhall et al. (1998:606) previously demonstrated that the 16-metre PACER test correlated well with VO_2 peak in children living with ID.

☐ Body mass index

This test is an important means to determine one's body mass relative to one's height. The test is easy to perform in the field setting and does not require sophisticated equipment. It has been reported that BMI is a reasonable index of adiposity with dual-energy X-ray absorptiometer measurements in adults living with ID (Temple, Walkley & Greenway 2010:116).

■ Percentile norms

Normative scores of functional fitness are provided when a study has assessed scores in a large epidemiological study. The data are summarised as descriptive statistics and represented as percentile tables. Norm-referenced percentile tables indicate the rank (0% – 100%) of a particular raw score. If one's score is associated with the 50th percentile in that specific test, it would mean that 50% of participants performed better and 50% performed worse. A percentile of 65% would mean that only 35% percent of participants performed better on that particular raw score. Norm-referenced percentile tables are provided in Chapter 3 according to gender and age categories (18-25; 26-35; 36-45; > 45) for adults living with DS. The tables presented were obtained from a large set of participants living with DS (n = 371) across seven provinces of South Africa. Data were obtained over a period of 6 months.

Although norm-referenced tables are provided, criterion-referenced tables are also important. As most adults living with DS have low functional fitness (Boer 2010:105), it is recommended to compare raw scores to a particular criterion rather than to normative tables (as the 50th percentile scores in these tables are too low to indicate optimal functional ability). For example, an individual living with DS might gain more information through the knowledge of his or her risk for developing physical disability or dependence in later years compared to the average score of individuals in his or her population. Consequently, Rikli and Jones (2013) developed criterion standards with cut-off points to indicate scores associated with independent and disability-free functioning in later years. However, both norm- and criterion-referenced tables provide important information regarding functional fitness. Norm-referenced tables allow a participant to compare his or her score to peers and to track his or her score over a period of time.

However, regarding independence in later years, criterion-referenced tables provide a preferable alternative. It is best to use longitudinal data combined with a composite physical function as used by Rikli and Jones (2013:43). Over time, a well-constructed longitudinal analysis of criterion-referenced standards will also be developed for the FFTB. In the interim, we recommend tentative scores of at or above the 75th percentile score as minimal optimal values (except for the two flexibility test items) until validated criterion-referenced scores are obtained for adults living with DS (Rikli & Jones 2013:43).

The BPFT also based some of their specific standards on expert opinion and related literature. The 75th percentile value was based on similar guidelines as suggested by the BPFT and experts in the field of DS. The value was chosen in the higher brackets of percentile norms (rather than medial values) to ensure and safeguard against future physical disabilities or other comorbidities. It is important to remember that these norm-referenced scores are presented for physically active and inactive participants and this should be considered by research and academic scholars when these tests are assessed. Therefore, physically active individuals will rate higher on the percentile norms. It should also be remembered that these norms are associated with individuals living with DS (the non-mosaic type). The non-mosaic type is the most frequent occurrence of DS (99% of all cases). Individuals living with mosaic DS (1% of cases) perform better on functional fitness tests and should not compare themselves to these normative tables.

■ Study results illustrating participant characteristics and percentile norms

The epidemiological study conducted by Terblanche and Boer (2013:830) provided large-scale information pertaining to the participant characteristics (total number of participants, age, height, body mass, BMI, sitting height and arm span) in their different categories (Table 3.5). Data for the percentile-based norms, categorised according to gender and age, are provided in this chapter for 11 of the 12 functional fitness tests. Currently, no percentile tables are available for the standardised 6-minute walk distance test. A percentile rank at the 50th percentile indicates that 50% of scores in that particular group obtained a better score. A percentile rank at the 25th percentile indicates that 75% of scores in that particular group obtained a better score.

TABLE 3.5: Descriptive statistics of adults with Down syndrome.

Categories	Participants	Age groups				
		Combined	18–25	26–35	36–45	> 45
Mean age (years)	Men	34.0 (10.4)	21.4 (2.4)	30.5 (3.1)	40.3 (3.0)	50.7 (3.8)
	Women	34.2 (10.7)	21.7 (2.2)	30.8 (3.0)	40.1 (3.0)	51.5 (5.3)
Height (cm) #	Men	158.3 (7.6)	157.6 (8.2)	157.6 (7.3)	158.8 (7.2)	159.8 (7.6)
	Women	146.8 (6.9)	147.4 (7.4)	147.4 (5.8)	147.6 (7.1)	143.6 (6.9)
Body mass (kg) # *	Men	74.6 (12.9)	76.1 (13.6)	76.6 (13.8)	72.6 (11.3)	72.1 (12.6)
	Women	68.6 (13.5)	69.2 (13.3)	68.1 (14.81)	71.5 (12.4)	63.9 (12.2)
Sitting height (cm) #	Men	84.8 (4.1)	84.3 (4.1)	85.2 (4.3)	85 (3.8)	84.4 (4.1)
	Women	79.3 (4.1)	80.5 (4.3)	80.0 (3.2)	79.5 (3.5)	75.9 (4.5)
Arm span (cm) # *	Men	156.9 (7.9)	156.6 (7.9)	155.8 (8.0)	157.6 (8.7)	158.3 (6.1)
	Women	143.5 (7.4)	144.6 (8.0)	143.8 (7.2)	142.9 (7.6)	141.9 (5.8)
BMI #	Men	29.9 (5.6)	30.8 (6.0)	30.1 (6.0)	28.9 (5.0)	28.2 (4.5)
	Women	31.9 (6.4)	32.0 (6.2)	31.4 (6.7)	33.1 (6.4)	31.1 (5.9)
Total no of participants	**Men**	**199**	**53**	**58**	**58**	**30**
	Women	**172**	**46**	**52**	**46**	**28**
	Total	**371**	**99**	**109**	**104**	**58**

Source: Terblanche and Boer (2013).
Note: BMI, Body Mass Index; *, $p < 0.01$ across age categories; #, $p < 0.01$ between gender.

■ Criterion-referenced standards

As explained in the section 'Study results illustrating participant characteristics and percentile norms', criterion-referenced tables provide important information pertaining to minimally acceptable standards. As most adults living with DS have low functional fitness (Boer 2010:78–86), it is recommended to compare raw scores to a particular criterion rather than to normative tables (as the 50th percentile scores in these tables are too low to indicate optimal functional ability). Rikli and Jones (2013:43) developed criterion standards with cut-off points to indicate scores associated with independent and disability-free functioning in later years. It is best to use longitudinal data combined with a composite physical function as used by Rikli and Jones (2013:43). The 12-item composite physical function scale was designed to assess physical function for ADL, instrumental ADL and more strenuous ADL.

A well-constructed longitudinal analysis of criterion-referenced standards will be developed for the FFTB in due course. In the interim, we recommend tentative scores of at or above the 75th percentile score as minimal optimal values (except for the two flexibility test items) until validated criterion-referenced scores are obtained for adults living with DS (Rikli & Jones 2013:43). The BPFT (Winnick & Short 2014:29) also based some of its specific standards on expert opinion and related literature. The 75th percentile value was based on similar guidelines as suggested by the BPFT and experts in the field of DS. The value was chosen in the higher brackets of percentile norms (rather than medial values) to ensure and safeguard against future physical disabilities or other comorbidities. It is also important to remember that these norm-referenced scores are presented for physically active and inactive participants and this should be considered by the academic scholar or exercise specialist when these tests are assessed. Therefore, physically active individuals will rate higher on the percentile norms. It should also be remembered that these norms are associated with individuals living with DS (the non-mosaic type). The non-mosaic type is the most frequent occurrence of DS (99% of all cases). Individuals with mosaic DS (1% of cases) perform better on functional fitness tests and should not compare themselves to these normative tables.

The following tables illustrate the norm- and criterion-referenced tables for the FFTB (Table 3.6 – Table 3.27):

1. Balance (Table 3.6 – Table 3.9).
2. Flexibility (Table 3.10 – Table 3.13).
3. Muscular strength and endurance (Table 3.14 – Table 3.23).
4. Functional ability (Table 3.24 – Table 3.25).
5. Aerobic capacity (Table 3.26 – Table 3.27).

TABLE 3.6: Balance-standing on one leg (seconds) – Men.

Percentile rank	18–25	26–35	36–45	> 45
95	10	10	10	10
90	10	10	10	10
85	10	10	10	10
80	10	10	10	8.7
75	10	10	10	7.7
70	10	10	10	5.6
65	10	10	8.8	5.0
60	10	10	7.0	4.4
55	10	10	6.0	3.8
50	9.1	7.2	5.4	3.6
45	8.2	6.6	5.0	2.9
40	7.0	5.8	3.8	2.6
35	6.6	5.5	3.4	2.3
30	4.6	3.6	2.8	2.0
25	3.1	3.2	2.6	1.5
20	2.6	2.0	2.3	1.4
15	1.9	1.8	1.5	1.2
10	1.4	1.4	1.3	0.9
5	1.0	0.9	0.7	0.4

Source: See Boer (2010).
Note: Values at the 75th percentile; bolded values are the criterion-referenced values.

TABLE 3.7: Balance-standing on one leg (seconds) – Women.

Percentile rank	18–25	26–35	36–45	> 45
95	10	10	10	10
90	10	10	10	8.3
85	10	10	10	6.3
80	10	10	9.0	6.0
75	**10**	**10**	**6.9**	**4.8**
70	10	10	4.8	3.2
65	8.4	10	3.8	2.9
60	7.4	7.4	3.3	2.5
55	6.9	5.5	3.1	2.3
50	5.1	4.3	2.6	1.7
45	4.2	3.5	2.4	1.5
40	2.7	3.0	2.3	1.4
35	2.6	3.0	2.2	1.1
30	2.4	2.4	2.0	0.9
25	1.9	1.8	1.5	0.8
20	1.8	1.6	1.4	0.6
15	1.5	1.4	1.2	0.5
10	1.2	1.3	1.2	0
5	1.2	0.8	1.0	0

Source: See Boer (2010).
Note: Values at the 75th percentile; bolded values are the criterion-referenced values.

TABLE 3.8: Balance – Walking on balance beam (steps) – Men.

Percentile rank	18–25	26–35	36–45	> 45
95	6	6	6	6
90	6	6	6	6
85	6	6	6	6
80	6	6	6	5
75	**6**	**6**	**6**	**4**
70	6	6	6	3.5
65	6	6	5	3
60	6	6	4	3
55	6	6	4	3
50	6	5	3	2.5
45	5	5	3	2
40	5	4	3	2
35	4	3	3	1
30	4	3	2	0.5
25	3	2	1	0
20	3	2	1	0
15	2	1	1	0
10	0	0	0	0
5	0	0	0	0

Source: See Boer (2010).
Note: Values at the 75th percentile; bolded values are the criterion-referenced values.

TABLE 3.9: Balance – Walking on balance beam (steps) – Women.

Percentile rank	18–25	26–35	36–45	> 45
95	6	6	6	6
90	6	6	6	6
85	6	6	6	4
80	6	6	5	4
75	**6**	**6**	**4**	**3**
70	6	6	4	0
65	6	6	3	0
60	6	6	3	0
55	6	5	2	0
50	5	4.5	2	0
45	4	4	2	0
40	3	3	2	0
35	3	2	1	0
30	3	1	1	0
25	2	1	0	0
20	1	1	0	0
15	0	0	0	0
10	0	0	0	0
5	0	0	0	0

Source: See Boer (2010).
Note: Values at the 75th percentile; bolded values are the criterion-referenced values.

TABLE 3.10: Flexibility – Back scratch (cm) – Men.

Percentile rank	18–25	26–35	36–45	> 45
95	11	13	10	9
90	8	8	8	7
85	8	6	5	4
80	7	5	4	3
75	6	4	3	0
70	5	2	2	–2.5
65	4	1	0	–3
60	3	0	–1	–4
55	2	–2	–2	–4
50	1	–4.5	–2	–6
45	–1	–6	–3	–7
40	**–5**	**–7**	**–4**	**–8**
35	–6	–10	–5	–8
30	–8	–13	–8	–10.5
25	–10	–13	–9	–13
20	–11	–15	–11	–13
15	–14	–16	–14	–17
10	–17	–20	–19	–17.5
5	–20	–27	–20	–24

Source: See Boer (2010).
Note: Values at the 40th percentile; bolded values are the criterion-referenced values.

TABLE 3.11: Flexibility – Back scratch (cm) – Women.

Percentile rank	18–25	26–35	36–45	> 45
95	6	6	4	3
90	5	4	3	3
85	5	4	2	2
80	4	3	2	2
75	4	2.5	1	−0.5
70	3	1	−1	−4
65	2	0	−5	−5
60	1	−2	−6	−5
55	0	−4	−8	−5
50	0	−6	−10	−7.5
45	−2	−7	−11	−8
40	**−2**	**−8**	**−12**	**−9**
35	−3	−8	−13	−10
30	−5	−10	−14	−10
25	−6	−11	−15	−13
20	−7	−12	−15	−14
15	−12	−14	−20	−17
10	−12	−18	−24	−17
5	−14	−25	−26	−20

Source: See Boer (2010).
Note: Values at the 40th percentile; bolded values are the criterion-referenced values.

TABLE 3.12: Flexibility – Chair sit–and–reach (cm) – Men.

Percentile rank	18–25	26–35	36–45	> 45
95	23	24	23	15
90	20	21	19	12.5
85	20	18	15	12
80	17	16	13	9.5
75	16	15	11	8
70	15	14	9	8
65	14	12	8	7
60	11	12	7	5.5
55	11	10	6	5
50	8	6.5	5	4.5
45	4	5	3	4
40	**3**	**4**	**1**	**2.5**
35	2	3	1	2
30	1	2	0	0
25	1	1.5	0	−2
20	0	1	−1	−3
15	−5	0	−5	−3
10	−5	−3.	−6	−7
5	−8	−8.	−13	−10

Source: See Boer (2010).
Note: Values at the 40th percentile; bolded values are the criterion–referenced values.

TABLE 3.13: Flexibility – Chair sit-and-reach (cm) – Women.

Percentile rank	18–25	26–35	36–45	> 45
95	22	20	18	14
90	19	16	15	13
85	17	14	15	13
80	16	13	14	12
75	15	12	12	10.5
70	15	11	10	9
65	13	10	8	9
60	12	10	7	8
55	12	10	6	7
50	11	9	5.5	7
45	10	8	5	6
40	**9**	**5**	**5**	**6**
35	7	4	3	4
30	5	3	0	4
25	4	2	−2	1.5
20	3	0	−2	−1
15	1	−1	−3	−3
10	−9	−3	−5	−3
5	−15	−7	−8	−5

Source: See Boer (2010).
Note: Values at the 40th percentile; bolded values are the criterion-referenced values.

TABLE 3.14: Muscular strength and endurance – 30-second chair stand test (number of stands) – Men.

Percentile rank	18–25	26–35	36–45	> 45
95	17	17	17	15
90	16	16	14	13
85	16	16	14	13
80	15	15	14	12
75	**15**	**14**	**13**	**12**
70	14	14	13	12
65	14	13	12	12
60	14	13	12	11
55	13	13	12	11
50	13	12.5	12	11
45	13	12	11	11
40	13	12	11	10
35	13	12	11	10
30	12	11	10	9.5
25	12	11	10	9
20	11	11	10	8.5
15	11	10	9	8
10	10	10	9	8
5	9	9	8	7

Source: See Boer (2010).
Note: Values at the 75th percentile; bolded values are the criterion-referenced values.

TABLE 3.15: Muscular strength and endurance – Chair stands (number of stands) – Women.

Percentile rank	18–25	26–35	36–45	> 45
95	16	18	16	15
90	16	16	15	15
85	16	15	15	14
80	15	15	14	14
75	**14**	**14.5**	**14**	**13**
70	14	14	13	13
65	14	14	13	12
60	13	13	13	12
55	13	13	13	11
50	13	12.5	12	11
45	12	12	12	11
40	12	12	12	11
35	12	12	11	10
30	11	11	11	9
25	11	11	11	8
20	11	11	11	8
15	10	10	10	8
10	9	10	9	7
5	8	9	9	7

Source: See Boer (2010).
Note: Values at the 75th percentile; bolded values are the criterion-referenced values.

TABLE 3.16: Muscular strength and endurance – Isometric push-up (seconds) – Men.

Percentile rank	18–25	26–35	36–45	> 45
95	138.6	153.6	108	86.8
90	104.0	97.0	87.0	73.0
85	88.0	80.6	81.0	59.3
80	85.0	77.1	75.2	51.3
75	**76.2**	**71.5**	**70.7**	**48.6**
70	70.0	66.5	66.5	44.6
65	66.5	58.0	65.9	41.5
60	64.8	56.8	57.1	35.7
55	60.0	53.7	50.4	26.5
50	50.7	48.0	49.0	25.0
45	45.1	47.0	45.0	24.5
40	42.7	40.0	40.6	21.6
35	40.0	33.7	39.5	16.8
30	34.0	32.7	38.1	11.6
25	32.4	24.4	35.0	11.0
20	23.1	18.9	29.9	9.4
15	20.8	8.0	16.6	8.2
10	20.0	6.0	4.0	5.4
5	13.0	1.0	0.0	0.0

Source: See Boer (2010).
Note: Values at the 75th percentile; bolded values are the criterion-referenced values.

TABLE 3.17: Muscular strength and endurance – Isometric push-up (seconds) – Women.

Percentile rank	18–25	26–35	36–45	> 45
95	71.0	87.0	56.8	66.4
90	61.4	72.0	49.2	59.2
85	56.1	69.2	46	53.4
80	50.6	54.9	40.8	41.1
75	**46.6**	**53.8**	**40.0**	**34.0**
70	45.0	51.9	38.1	30.8
65	40.0	42.0	34.6	23.5
60	38.4	40.0	28.9	18.7
55	34.0	34.0	27.0	16.8
50	30.6	33.0	24.6	11.6
45	21.9	32.2	23.1	6.5
40	18.8	23.0	20.6	5.2
35	13.7	22.2	19.0	0.0
30	10.3	21.0	10.7	0.0
25	9.5	15.7	9.0	0.0
20	8.0	13.0	2.6	0.0
15	4.1	8.7	0.0	0.0
10	0.0	3.4	0.0	0.0
5	0.0	1.2	0.0	0.0

Source: See Boer (2010).
Note: Values at the 75th percentile; bolded values are the criterion-referenced values.

TABLE 3.18: Muscular strength and endurance – Handgrip strength (kg) – Men.

Percentile rank	18–25	26–35	36–45	> 45
95	45.1	44.3	41.9	41.9
90	38.3	40.4	41.1	41.6
85	36.9	40.0	38.7	38.9
80	35.9	39.0	34.9	37.5
75	**34.9**	**38.0**	**33.9**	**36.3**
70	34.4	37.1	33.1	34.0
65	33.6	35.1	32.3	31.3
60	33.6	33.9	31.1	30.5
55	32.9	33.4	30.0	28.3
50	31.1	31.6	29.9	27.1
45	29.3	30.3	29.0	26.7
40	28.9	29.7	27.1	25.8
35	27.9	27.9	26.1	23.9
30	26.0	25.7	25.3	23.3
25	25.7	25.0	24.2	22.9
20	23.1	23.2	22.9	21.8
15	20.8	21.4	21.3	19.7
10	19.2	16.1	19.2	19.4
5	14.8	10.6	13.2	18.6

Source: See Boer (2010).
Note: Values at the 75th percentile; bolded values are the criterion-referenced values.

TABLE 3.19: Muscular strength and endurance – Handgrip strength (kg) – Women.

Percentile rank	18–25	26–35	36–45	> 45
95	27.5	32.6	30	29.7
90	26.8	27.5	27.2	25.8
85	26.4	26.5	26.7	24.6
80	25.0	24.6	25.6	23.2
75	**23.9**	**24.2**	**25**	**22.7**
70	23.8	23.5	23.8	22.1
65	22.6	22.5	23.2	21.7
60	22.1	22.2	22.7	21.0
55	21.5	21.5	22.2	20.1
50	21.3	21.1	21.5	18.4
45	20.3	20.7	21.3	17.5
40	19.7	20.4	20.4	17.5
35	19.3	20.0	20.0	15.6
30	18.3	18.2	18.0	15.4
25	17.2	18.0	16.8	14.5
20	16.6	17.7	16.4	12.0
15	15.5	17.2	13.8	11.8
10	14.1	16.2	12.7	9.4
5	12.1	13.9	12.1	8.4

Source: See Boer (2010).
Note: Values at the 75th percentile; bolded values are the criterion-referenced values.

TABLE 3.20: Muscular strength and endurance – Modified curl-up (number) – Men.

Percentile rank	18–25	26–35	36–45	> 45
95	75	75	75	75
90	75	75	75	37.5
85	75	68	75	30
80	75	54	41	23.5
75	**54**	**35**	**34**	**19**
70	50	26	30	16.5
65	38	22	25	11
60	31	13	22	8.5
55	31	11	16	5
50	17	7.5	12	2
45	10	6	8	0
40	8	4	6	0
35	3	3	1	0
30	1	0	0	0
25	0	0	0	0
20	0	0	0	0
15	0	0	0	0
10	0	0	0	0
5	0	0	0	0

Source: See Boer (2010).
Note: Values at the 75th percentile; bolded values are the criterion-referenced values.

TABLE 3.21: Muscular strength and endurance – Modified curl-up (number) – Women.

Percentile rank	18-25	26-35	36-45	> 45
95	75	75	32.0	50
90	65	75	25	36
85	35	64	23	3
80	29	35	20.5	1
75	**20**	**31.5**	**19**	**0**
70	13	23	15	0
65	5	20	13	0
60	1	17	9	0
55	0	11	5	0
50	0	5.5	3	0
45	0	3	2	0
40	0	0	1	0
35	0	0	0	0
30	0	0	0	0
25	0	0	0	0
20	0	0	0	0
15	0	0	0	0
10	0	0	0	0
5	0	0	0	0

Source: See Boer (2010).
Note: Values at the 75th percentile; bolded values are the criterion-referenced values.

TABLE 3.22: Muscular strength and endurance – Trunk lift (cm) – Men.

Percentile rank	18-25	26-35	36-45	> 45
95	44	46	42	35
90	41	42	39	34.5
85	37	41	37	32
80	36	39	36	29.5
75	**34**	**39**	**34**	**29**
70	34	38	34	29
65	33	37	32	27
60	31	35	32	26
55	31	33	31	25
50	30	32.5	30	23.5
45	29	30	30	22
40	29	28	28	19
35	28	28	28	17
30	26	27	27	16.5
25	25	26	26	16
20	23	24	25	16
15	20	22	21	14
10	20	20	18	12
5	13	16	14	10

Source: See Boer (2010).
Note: Values at the 75th percentile; bolded values are the criterion-referenced values.

TABLE 3.23: Muscular strength and endurance – Trunk lift (cm) – Women.

Percentile rank	18–25	26–35	36–45	> 45
95	41	38	34	35
90	38	37	31	33
85	37	36	31	29
80	35	35	29.5	27
75	**34**	**33**	**29**	**26**
70	33	31	27	25
65	32	31	27	24
60	32	30	26	23
55	30	29	25	21
50	29	29	25	20
45	28	27	25	20
40	28	27	23.5	19
35	27	26	21	18
30	27	25	21	18
25	25	23.5	20	16
20	24	23	18.5	15
15	21	21	17	14
10	20	21	16	12
5	18	19	12	11

Source: See Boer (2010).
Note: Values at the 75th percentile; bolded values are the criterion-referenced values.

TABLE 3.24: Functional ability – 8-foot up-and-go (seconds) – Men.

Percentile rank	18–25	26–35	36–45	> 45
95	8.2	8.5	9.2	10.9
90	7.5	7.5	8.3	9.3
85	7.3	7.2	7.7	8.5
80	6.8	6.9	7.6	8.2
75	**6.6**	**6.7**	**6.9**	**8.1**
70	6.4	6.5	6.6	7.8
65	6.0	6.2	6.5	7.1
60	5.9	6.0	6.4	7.0
55	5.8	5.9	6.2	6.9
50	5.6	5.9	6.1	6.8
45	5.5	5.9	5.9	6.7
40	5.3	5.7	5.7	6.6
35	5.1	5.6	5.6	6.3
30	4.9	5.4	5.5	6.2
25	4.9	5.2	5.2	6.0
20	4.8	5.1	5.0	5.8
15	4.5	4.9	4.9	5.4
10	4.4	4.4	4.7	5.4
5	4.2	4.3	4.6	4.8

Source: See Boer (2010).
Note: Values at the 75th percentile; bolded values are the criterion-referenced values.

TABLE 3.25: Functional ability – 8-foot up-and-go (seconds) – Women.

Percentile rank	18–25	26–35	36–45	> 45
95	7.9	7.9	9.8	13.5
90	7.7	7.7	8.8	12.8
85	7.4	7.2	8.6	11.6
80	6.9	6.7	8.4	10.0
75	**6.6**	**6.6**	**7.6**	**9.5**
70	6.5	6.5	7.4	9.1
65	6.3	6.4	7.2	8.5
60	6.2	6.3	7.1	7.9
55	6.0	6.2	6.7	7.8
50	5.8	6.1	6.5	7.5
45	5.7	6.0	6.3	7.3
40	5.7	5.7	6.2	7.3
35	5.6	5.6	6.1	7.0
30	5.5	5.4	6.0	7.0
25	5.2	5.3	5.8	6.5
20	5.1	5.2	5.6	6.2
15	5.0	5.1	5.5	6.0
10	4.9	4.9	5.3	5.4
5	4.8	4.5	5.0	5.1

Source: See Boer (2010).
Note: Values at the 75th percentile; bolded values are the criterion-referenced values.

TABLE 3.26: Aerobic capacity – 16-metre PACER (number of shuttles) – Men.

Percentile rank	18–25	26–35	36–45	> 45
95	57	56	47	31
90	42	52	33	25
85	42	42	32	20
80	35	34	30	16
75	**31**	**31**	**26**	**16**
70	30	27	25	15
65	26	25	22	13
60	26	24	19	12
55	24	21	17	12
50	24	19	16	11
45	23	17	14	11
40	21	15	13	9.5
35	18	14	11	7
30	17	12	11	7
25	15	12	10	4
20	13	8	10	3
15	11	8	8	3
10	11	7	7	2.5
5	5	3	5	1

Source: See Boer (2010).
Note: Values at the 75th percentile; bolded values are the criterion-referenced values.

TABLE 3.27: Aerobic capacity – 16-metre PACER (number of shuttles) – Women.

Percentile rank	18–25	26–35	36–45	> 45
95	27	38	20	15
90	23	23	16	13
85	22	21	15	13
80	21	19	14	13
75	**18**	**15**	**14**	**9.5**
70	17	15	12	9
65	16	15	10	8
60	16	13	10	6
55	15	13	10	6
50	15	12	9	5
45	13	11	9	5
40	12	11	8	4
35	11	11	8	4
30	10	10	8	3
25	10	8	7	1.5
20	8	8	5	1
15	6	7	4	0
10	3	7	3	0
5	1	7	2	0

Source: See Boer (2010).
Note: Values at the 75th percentile; bolded values are the criterion-referenced values.

■ Summary

In summary, based on the large epidemiological study performed on adults living with DS (Terblanche & Boer 2013:826) and the test-retest reliability and validity (Boer & Moss 2016b:176, 2016c:2575) and the criterion, discriminant and logical validity provided by academic scholars and other researchers working in the field of adapted physical activity or elderly individuals, we believe that there is sufficient evidence for using the functional fitness battery for adults living with DS to assess functional fitness.

Test administration

■ Pre-test procedures

Testing venue

The testing venue should be prepared before testing can take place. Ensure that a spacious room or hall that is free from noise or disturbances is used. The temperature in the testing venue should not be too hot or too cold (ideally 18 °C – 25 °C). The surface of the testing room should be non-slippery. The stations for all 12 functional fitness tests should be prepared according to the details presented in the full descriptions of the functional fitness tests. Table 4.1 provides an overview of the equipment needed for the FFTB. A detailed breakdown is provided for each test in the latter part of this chapter (full description of the FFTB).

Pre-test screening

Prior to testing, the participant has to visit his or her primary physician to determine whether he or she is able to perform physical activity. The adapted physical activity readiness questionnaire (app. G) should be completed by the

How to cite: Boer, P.-H., 2021, 'Test administration', in *Functional fitness for adults living with Down syndrome*, pp. 47–64, AOSIS, Cape Town. https://doi.org/10.4102/aosis.2021.BK252.04

TABLE 4.1: Equipment needed for the functional fitness test battery.

Test items	Equipment
General	Pen, recording sheet, clipboard, stopwatch, cones, 50-cm steel ruler and measuring table (20 m and 5 m)
Body mass and height	Calibrated electronic scale, 150-cm tape measure, prestic and steel ruler
Standing on one leg	Stopwatch
Walking on balance beam	Balance beam (3.05 m in length and 10.16 cm wide)
Back scratch	50-cm steel ruler
Chair sit-and-reach	50-cm steel ruler and 43-cm folding chair
Chair stands (cm)	Stopwatch and 43-cm folding chair
Isometric push-up	Gymnasium mat and stopwatch
Handgrip strength	Handgrip strength dynamometer and 43-cm folding chair
Modified curl-up	Gymnasium mat
Trunk lift	Gymnasium mat and 50-cm steel ruler
8-foot up-and-go	Stopwatch, 43-cm folding chair and 5-m tape measure and cone
6-minute walk distance	Stopwatch and 4 cones
16-metre PACER	CD player, 4 cones, 20-m tape measure and PACER test CD

physician. Many adults living with DS are born with heart disease and should refrain from strenuous activities (especially the 16-metre PACER test).

Informed consent

The participant and parent/guardian should sign an information sheet and consent form (whether for research purposes or private use) to ensure that the purpose, nature, risks, individual rights and responsibilities of functional fitness testing are understood (app. A).

Person administering the test

The person administering the test should be qualified as a research scholar or adapted physical activity specialist and have experience in working with adults living with DS. Knowledge and experience in adapted physical activity is important. It must be remembered that adults living with DS have many conditions contraindicative to exercise and their motivational levels are not of the highest calibre. Therefore, the person administering the test should be an experienced academic or research scholar.

Pre-test instructions to the participants

To ensure reliable and maximal testing, participants should follow these basic instructions before the test day (This information is also provided in app. B):

- No strenuous physical activity for 24 h prior to testing.
- No alcohol or caffeine consumption for 24 h prior to testing.

- A light meal should be eaten 1h prior to testing.
- The bladder should be voided before testing.
- Light clothes and appropriate shoes should be worn on testing day.
- The completed informed consent and adapted physical activity readiness questionnaire must accompany the participant on testing day.

Data scoresheets

Forms for recording of test results can be prepared the day before exercise testing. They are available in Appendix E. An example is also presented in this chapter.

Warm-up

Warming-up is an essential activity for exercise testing. It raises the temperature of the body, increases the heart rate, gets the blood flowing and prepares all physiological mechanisms important for exercise. As a result, the chance of injury decreases.

The warm-up should last for about 5 min to 10 min. Any activities where the larger muscle groups are stressed is permissible. However, the activity should not be too strenuous. Walking 200 m or marching in place, swinging the arms, dancing to music (individuals with DS are known to love music) are all examples of a warm-up. A few stretches, especially the areas that will be tested during the assessment (hamstring and shoulders) are also important. A few examples are calf stretches, hamstring stretches, arm stretches, shoulder stretches, and head and neck stretches. The warm-up should precede the stretching. Stretching should be performed slowly and gradually, without bouncing or jerking movements.

Equipment

See Appendix C for all equipment required for the FFTB. The 'Full description of functional fitness testing' explains which tests are associated with what equipment.

Important general information and safety instructions when testing adults living with Down syndrome

Adults living with DS have an ID. As discussed previously, only adults who are able to understand test instructions and procedures are eligible for participation. The instructor should demonstrate slowly and use simple easy-to-understand words when explaining a specific test. The instructor should proceed by demonstrating the test at a normal pace to reiterate the importance of a timed test.

Adults living with DS have lower motivational levels. Thus the test battery was developed for a 1:1 (one instructor with one participant) testing ratio. Moreover, the instructor should continually motivate the participant to perform to his or her ability. Music is often a very helpful tool for adults living with DS.

Adults living with DS have to consult their primary physicians before exercise testing. A registered nurse or other health professional should be present when the two aerobic items are administered. If the participant experiences any pain (including chest pain), irregular heartbeat, dizziness or nausea, the testing should stop immediately (as described in pre-test procedures). The test should also be stopped if improper technique is used.

■ The full description of the functional fitness tests

An appendix is attached providing the key points for using this FFTB (app. H).

▪ General

This section provides a thorough summary of the purpose, equipment needed, procedure and scoring of all 14 functional fitness items. Before assessment, the instructor should demonstrate and slowly talk through the test before administration. The instructor should also demonstrate the timed tests in a faster motion to ensure that participants understand the nature of the test.

It is best if testing takes place between 08:00 and 11:00 to ensure uniformity. Testing should accrue in a spacious room or hall with a moderate temperature. Ideal testing conditions would be 18 °C – 25 °C.

Signs to stop testing or of overexertion include (but are not limited to):

- Chest pain
- Irregular heartbeat
- Any pain
- Nausea or vomiting
- Confusion
- Dizziness
- Loss of balance
- Blurred vision.

Testing should be implemented on a one-on-one basis. The test instructor should continually motivate all participants to perform to the best of their abilities. During the 6-minute walk distance test and the 6-metre PACER test, an instructor should walk or run alongside the participant for the entire duration of the test.

To minimise fatigue, it is recommended that the tests are organised in the following order (Boer & Moss 2016b:178): Flexibility items, 8-foot up-and-go, balance items, muscular strength and endurance (modified curl-up, trunk lift, 30-seconds chair stand, handgrip strength and isometric push-up), and finally the 6-minute walk distance test (see Boer 2015). A 5 min break should be provided between all tests. The 6-metre PACER test should be performed on the following day. The order of testing is provided in Appendix D.

Test items

Aerobic endurance

6-minute walk distance test

Purpose: To assess aerobic endurance whilst walking.

Equipment: Cones, measuring tape and stopwatch.

Procedure: The participant walks as fast as possible in a rectangle with a perimeter of 50 yards (20 yards by 5 yards) for 6 min. This is 18.23 m by 4.57 m. For improved accuracy and pacing, participants should practice this activity on the day before the test. On the signal 'go', the participant attempts to walk as many laps as possible within 6 min. No running is allowed. To assist with pacing, participants should be alerted every time a minute has elapsed.

Scoring: Convert the number of laps walked (rounded to the nearest quarter, half, three quarters or full lap) to the distance in yards or metres. One yard is 0.914 m. Only one trial is administered.

Safety precautions and general instructions: Stop the test if pain, dizziness, chest pain, heart palpitations or any sign or symptom contraindicated to exercise is experienced. Motivation is key. No running is allowed.

16-metre PACER test

Purpose: To assess aerobic endurance (running) (see Figure 4.1).

Equipment: Cones, measuring tape, CD player and PACER CD.

Procedure: At the sound of a tape-recorded beep, participants run from one line (cone) to the other, which should be 16 m away. If the participant fails to reach the line before the beep, a warning is provided. If he/she fails to reach

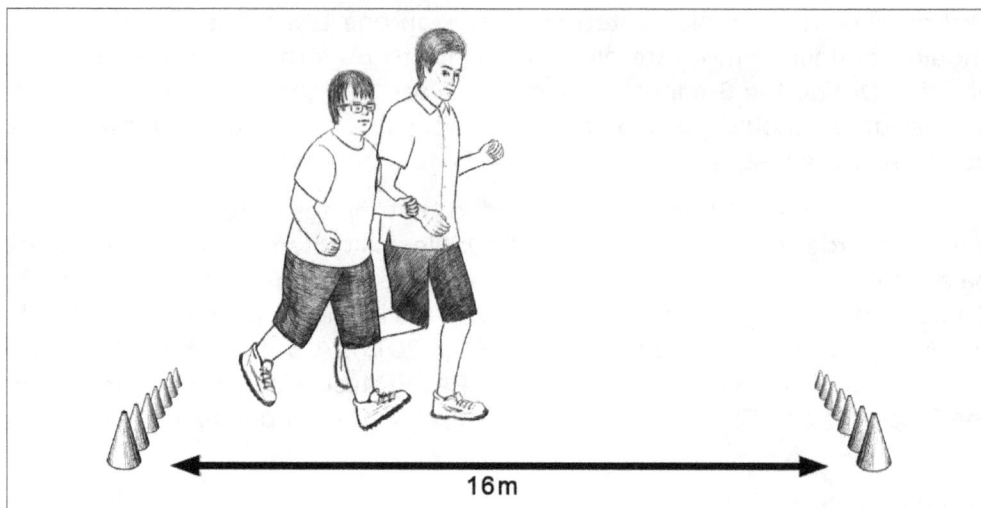

Source: Drawing published with permission from the artist, Luibov Mazanko, c. 2013-2015, Port Elizabeth, South Africa.
FIGURE 4.1: 16-metre PACER test.

the line again, the test is stopped. Only one trial is allowed. The test instructor should run alongside the participant (1:1 PACER). The sound of the tape-recorded beep increases in pace as the test progresses.

Scoring: The test score is the number of laps completed at the required pace.

Safety precautions and general instructions: Stop the test if pain, dizziness, chest pain, heart palpitations or any sign or symptom contraindicated to exercise is experienced. It is advised that a health professional is present during this test. Motivation is key. Ensure that the participant does not lose his/her balance during running or turning. Monitor participants for overexertion.

☐ Musculoskeletal functioning: Flexibility

☐ Chair sit-and-reach test

Purpose: To assess lower body flexibility (see Figure 4.2).

Equipment: Folding chair with a seat height of 43 cm (17 inches) with legs that angle forward to prevent tipping. A steel ruler of at least 50 cm. The chair is placed against the wall.

Procedure: This test is performed twice, first with one leg and then the other. The leg is extended straight in front of the hip, with the heel on the floor and the ankle flexed at 90° (the other leg is bent to the side with the foot flat on the floor). With the hands overlapped and the middle fingers even and on the

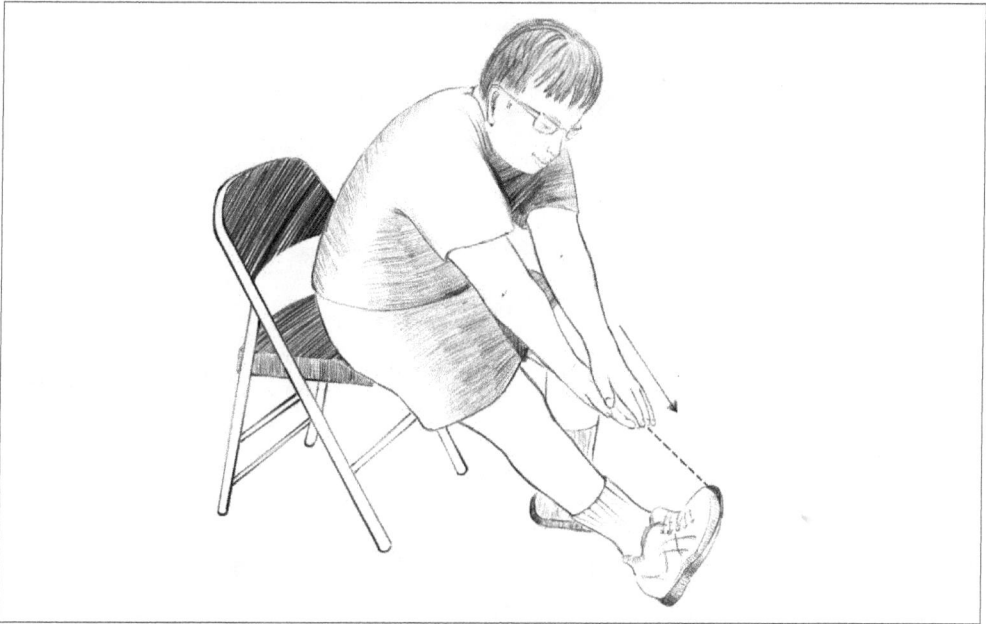

Source: Drawing published with permission from the artist, Luibov Mazanko, *c.* 2013-2015, Port Elizabeth, South Africa.
FIGURE 4.2: Chair sit-and-reach test.

steel ruler, the participant reaches as far as possible towards the toes (see Boer 2015). The maximum reach height must be held for at least 2 s. The same procedure is followed with the other leg. The instructor places one hand with the steel ruler on the participant's knee to ensure that there is no knee bend. The instructor's other hand is on the participant's toe and also holding the steel ruler.

Scoring: Two practice trials are allowed and two test trials on each leg. If the tip of the middle finger did not touch the toe, the distance short of the middle toe is measured and recorded as a negative score. If a middle finger reaches beyond the toes, the distance of overlap is measured and recorded as a positive score. The best valid attempt is regarded as the score.

Safety and general instructions: Place the chair against the wall. The participant should exhale as he or she stretches. No bouncing movements are allowed. Do not administer the test to participants with knee or hip injuries or who experience pain. The tested leg must remain extended.

Back scratch test

Purpose: To assess upper body (shoulder) flexibility (see Figure 4.3).

Equipment: 50-cm steel ruler.

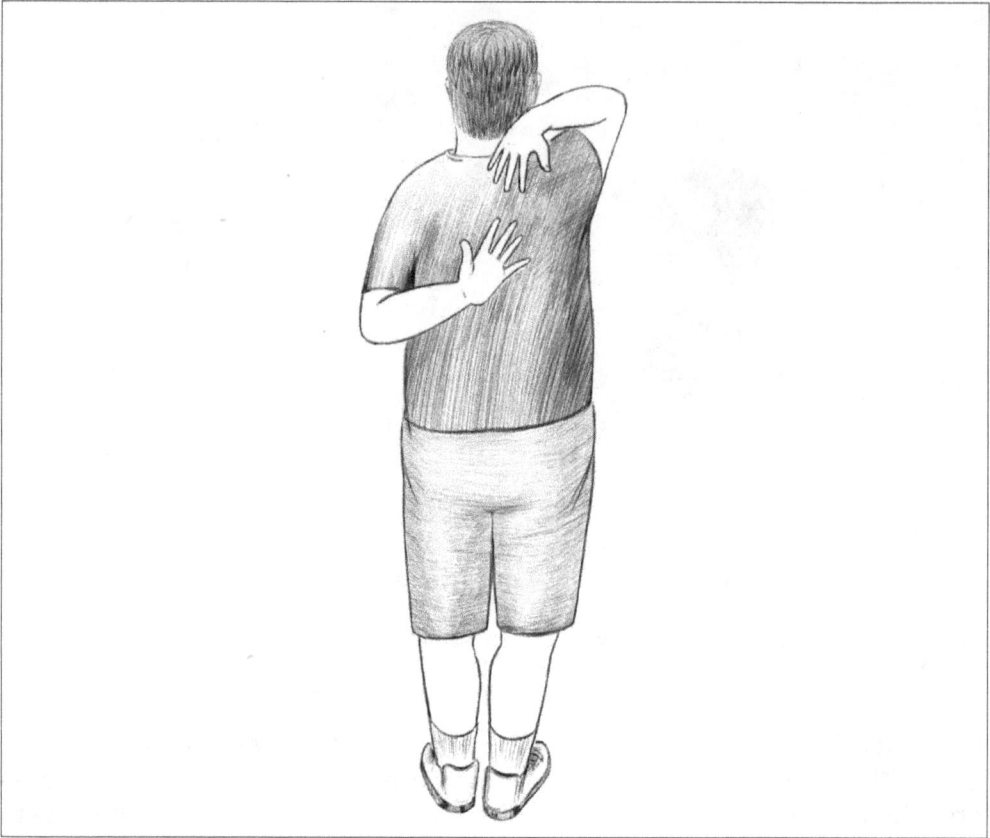

Source: Drawing published with permission from the artist, Luibov Mazanko, *c.* 2013-2015, Port Elizabeth, South Africa.
FIGURE 4.3: Back scratch test.

Procedure: Participants attempt to touch the fingertips of their two hands behind their backs. The participant reaches with his or her right hand in external rotation over the right shoulder between the scapulae, whilst the left elbow is bent, internally rotated and reaches upwards from the waist. Direct the participant's middle fingers towards each other without helping the stretch. The test is performed on the left and right side. In both tests, two practice trials are permissible. Two test trials are performed and the best score is noted. The maximum stretch should be held for at least 2 s.

Scoring: If the middle fingers of the two hands did not touch, the distance is measured and recorded as a negative score. If the middle fingers overlap, the distance of overlap is recorded as a positive score.

Safety and general instructions: Stop the test if the participant experiences pain. The participant should exhale as he or she stretches. No bouncing movements are allowed.

☐ Muscular strength and endurance

☐ Handgrip strength

Purpose: To assess forearm and handgrip strength (see Figure 4.4).

Equipment: Handgrip dynamometer, folding chair with no armrests.

Procedure: Handgrip strength is assessed by a grip dynamometer with a grip space of 10 cm. The dynamometer must be set to the size of the hand of the participant. The participant sits on a straight-backed chair without arms, with feet flat on the floor. The elbow is flexed at 90° and the grip dynamometer is squeezed as hard as possible. Three trials are administered, with 30 s rest between each trial. Both hands are tested. The best score for each hand is recorded.

Scoring: The device digitally records the participant's test score (kg).

☐ Isometric push-up

Purpose: To assess upper body endurance (see Figure 4.5).

Equipment: Stopwatch.

Procedure: Participants attempt to hold the push-up position for as long as they can. Hands are placed directly below the shoulders with arms extended.

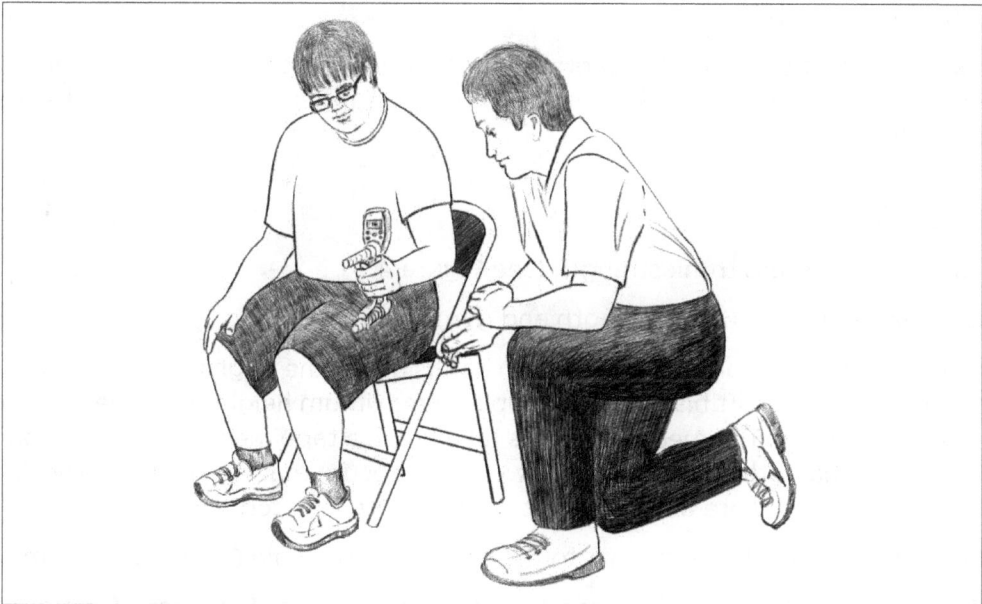

Source: Drawing published with permission from the artist, Luibov Mazanko, c. 2013-2015, Port Elizabeth, South Africa.
FIGURE 4.4: Handgrip strength.

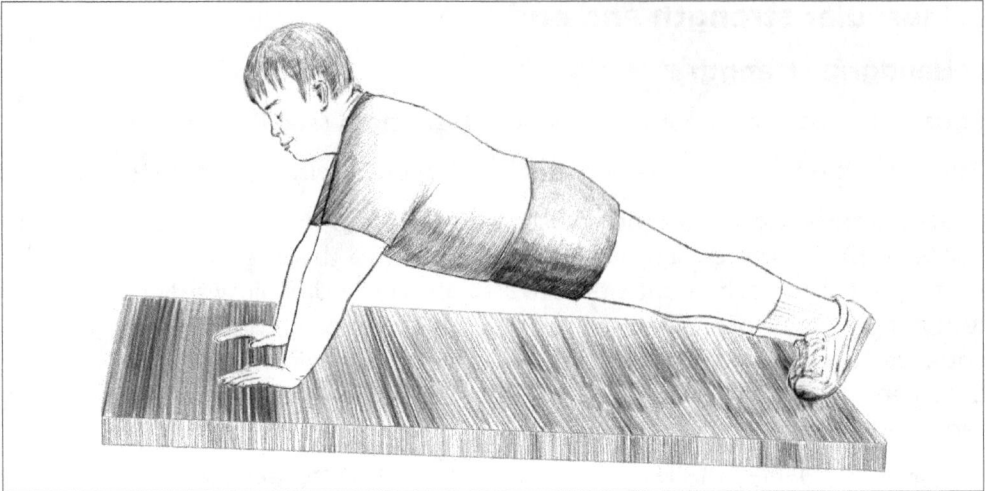

Source: Drawing published with permission from the artist, Luibov Mazanko, *c.* 2013-2015, Port Elizabeth, South Africa.
FIGURE 4.5: Isometric push-up.

The back has to be perfectly aligned with the rest of the body, and the toes have to be on the floor. The time that the position is held is recorded to the nearest second. Only one trial is administered. A practice session of 3 s to 5 s may be attempted to ensure proper posture. Time is stopped as soon as the back sags or lifts. Proper form is to be strictly controlled.

Scoring: Amount of time (in seconds) that the proper form of the push-up position is maintained.

Safety precautions and general instructions: Stop the test if pain is experienced. Motivation is key. Proper form (no sagging or lifting of the back) is important.

☐ Trunk lift

Purpose: To assess trunk strength (see Figure 4.6).

Equipment: Ruler 50 cm in length and gymnasium mat.

Procedure: From a prone position with hands under the thighs, the participant should attempt to lift his or her chin up to a maximum height from the mat by arching the back. The measurement is taken with a tape measure or ruler from the mat to the bottom of the chin (lower jaw). Ensure that the ruler is vertically straight. Two trials are allowed and the best score is noted.

Scoring: Distance from the mat to the bottom of the chin (lower jaw) in cm.

Safety precautions and general instructions: Stop the test if pain is experienced. Ensure that the hands remain under the thighs.

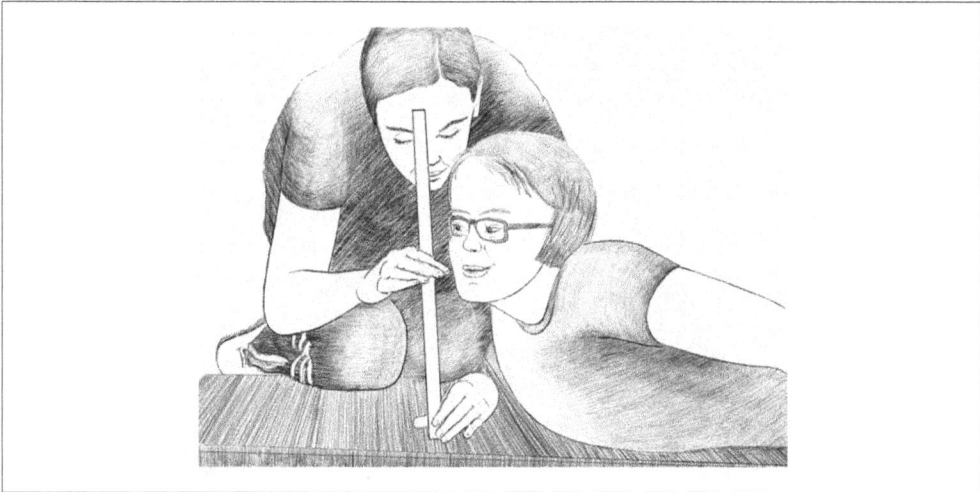

Source: Drawing published with permission from the artist, Luibov Mazanko, c. 2013-2015, Port Elizabeth, South Africa.
FIGURE 4.6: Trunk lift.

☐ Modified curl-up

Purpose: To assess abdominal strength and endurance (see Figure 4.7).

Equipment: Gymnasium mat.

Procedure: The participant lies in a supine position with knees bent and feet flat on the floor, with hands on the thighs. During the curl-up, the participant slides his or her hands up the thighs to the superior part of the kneecap and then returns to the starting position. The fingers have to slide at least 10 cm along the legs to the kneecaps. The instructor's hands should be placed on the superior aspect of the kneecap, thereby assisting the participant to perform the correct technique. Fingers are not allowed to lift off the legs and the hands have to slide simultaneously to the left and right kneecap (one hand should not lead the other). The participant should perform as many curl-ups as possible (a maximum of 75). The rate or pace of the curl-ups should be one curl-up every 3 s. The instructor should verbally count the number of curl-ups. Only one trial is administered. A practice trial of less than three curl-ups should be implemented.

Scoring: Number of curl-ups from starting position to the superior aspect of the knee cap.

Safety precautions and general instructions: Stop the test if pain is experienced. Ensure that the hands remain on the thighs throughout the movement. Hands should move up simultaneously. Motivation is key.

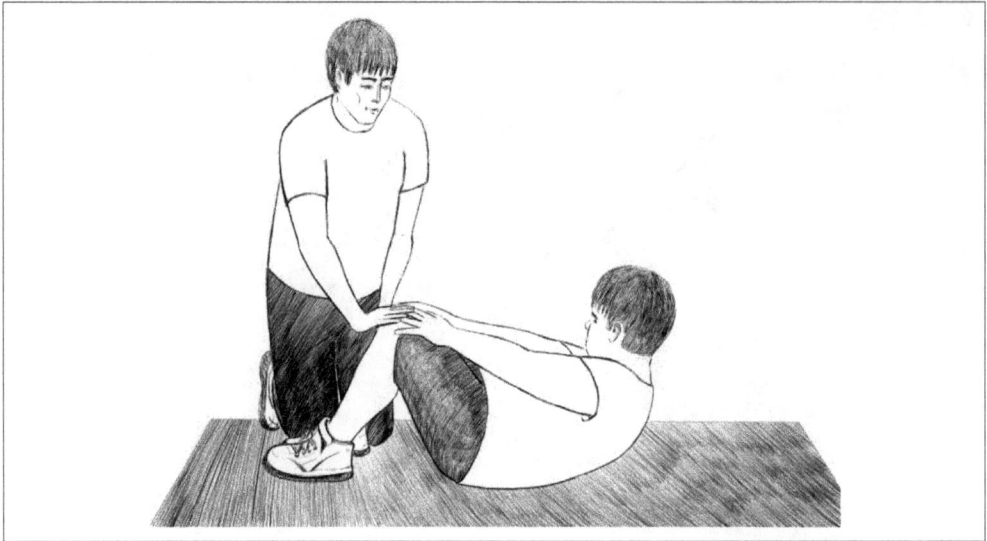

Source: Drawing published with permission from the artist, Luibov Mazanko, *c.* 2013-2015, Port Elizabeth, South Africa.
FIGURE 4.7: Modified curl-up.

☐ 30-second chair stand test

Purpose: To assess lower body strength (see Figure 4.8).

Equipment: Folding chair with a seat height of 43 cm (17 inches) and stopwatch.

Procedure: Participant sits on a straight-backed chair (43 cm in height and with no armrests), feet flat on the floor and arms across the chest. On the signal 'go', the participant rises to a full stand, and returns to a fully seated position. Before testing, the participant performs two or three stands to ensure correct technique. Every time the person sits, the back (positioned upright and straight) should touch the back of the chair. Two trials are administered.

Scoring: 'The score is the number of stands completed in 30 s. If the person is more than halfway up at the end of the 30 s, it is noted as a full stand' (see Saunders 2017).

Safety precautions and general instructions: Place the chair against the wall to prevent falling. Stand close to the chair in case the participant loses his or her balance. Stop the test if pain is experienced. Motivation is key.

☐ Balance

☐ Standing on one leg (stalk stand)

Purpose: To assess static balance (see Figure 4.9).

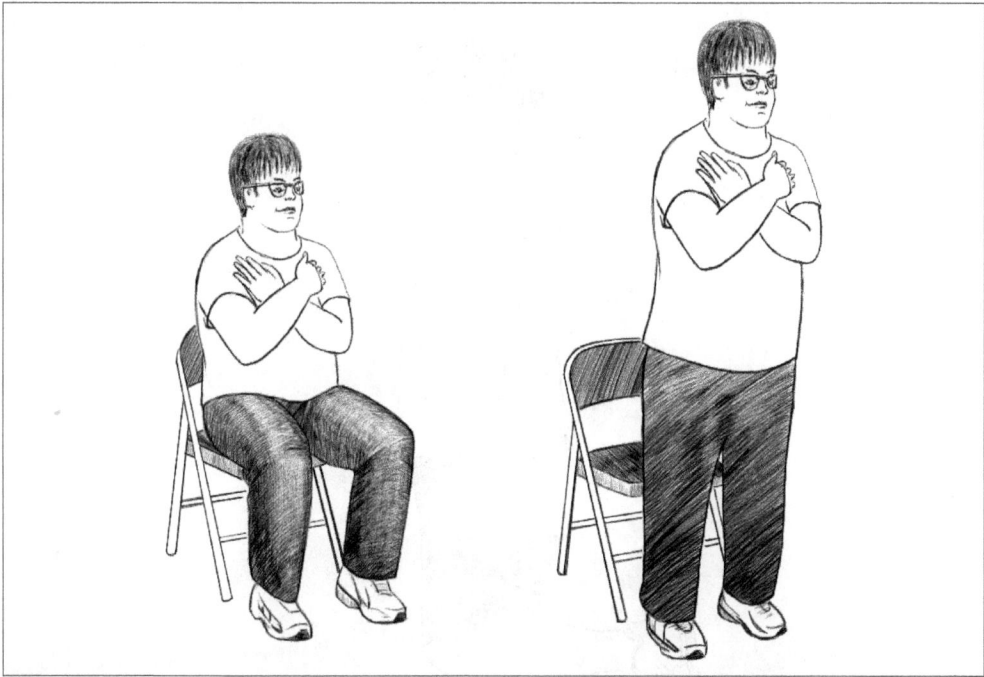

Source: Drawing published with permission from the artist, Luibov Mazanko, c. 2013-2015, Port Elizabeth, South Africa.
FIGURE 4.8: 30-second chair stand test.

Equipment: Stopwatch.

Procedure: This test assesses participant's ability to stand on one leg for as long as he or she can with a maximum time of 10 s. No shoes are allowed. The participant looks straight ahead with his or her hands on the hips. The knee of the free leg is fully bent so the lower leg is parallel to the floor. The knee or lower part of the bent leg may not touch the standing leg. The test is performed with both legs and the best score of each leg is noted as static balance performance. Two practice trials and two test trials on each leg are administered. The best score is noted.

Scoring: The test is terminated once the hands move off the hips and if too much body sway occurs.

Safety precautions and general instructions: Stop the test if the participant experiences pain. Stand next to the participant in case he or she loses balance.

☐ Walking on the balance beam

Purpose: To assess dynamic balance (see Figure 4.10).

Equipment: Balance beam (3.05 m by 10.16 cm).

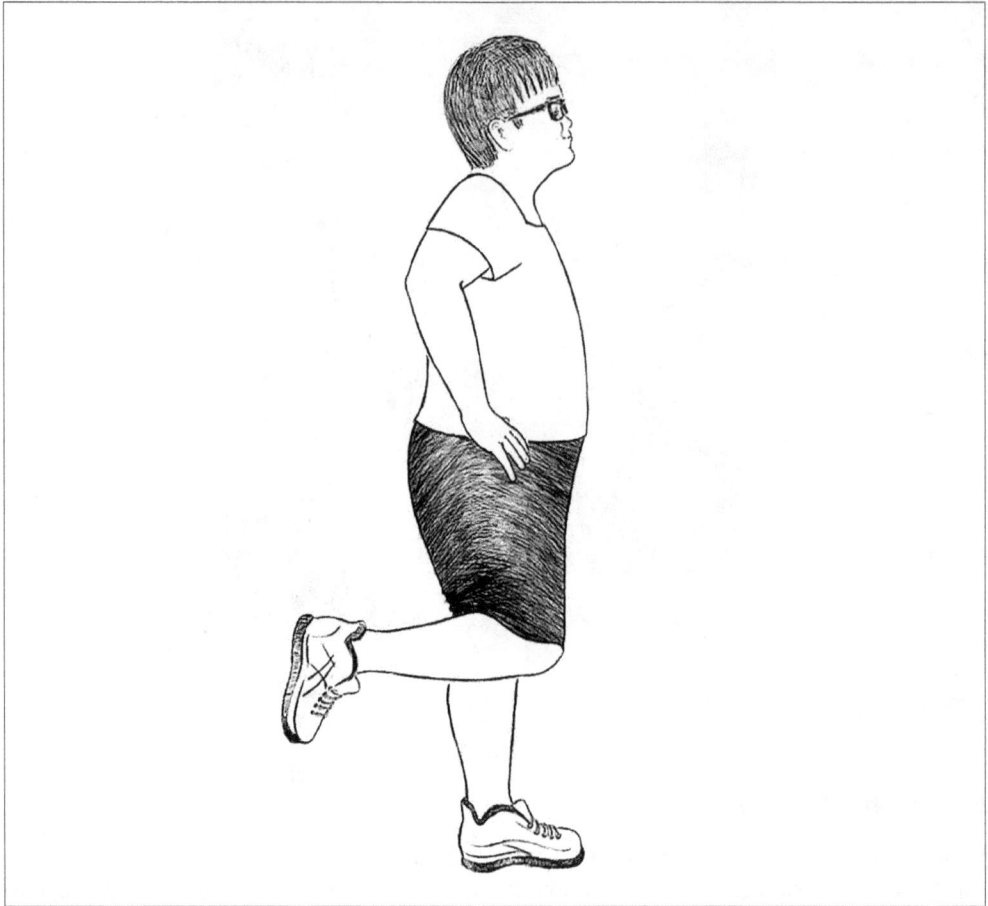

Source: Drawing published with permission from the artist, Luibov Mazanko, c. 2013-2015, Port Elizabeth, South Africa.
FIGURE 4.9: Standing on one leg.

Procedure: The participant is instructed to walk with a normal stride, with hands on the hips, across the balance beam. The number of consecutive steps completed on the balance beam, up to a maximum of six steps, is recorded. Two practise trials and two test trials are administered. The best score is noted.

Scoring: Amount of steps (maximum score is six).

Safety precautions and general instructions: Walk alongside the participant in case he or she loses balance. Both hands must remain on the hips. Participant may not take 'baby steps'.

☐ Functional test

☐ 8-foot up-and-go test

Purpose: To assess functional ability (see Figure 4.11).

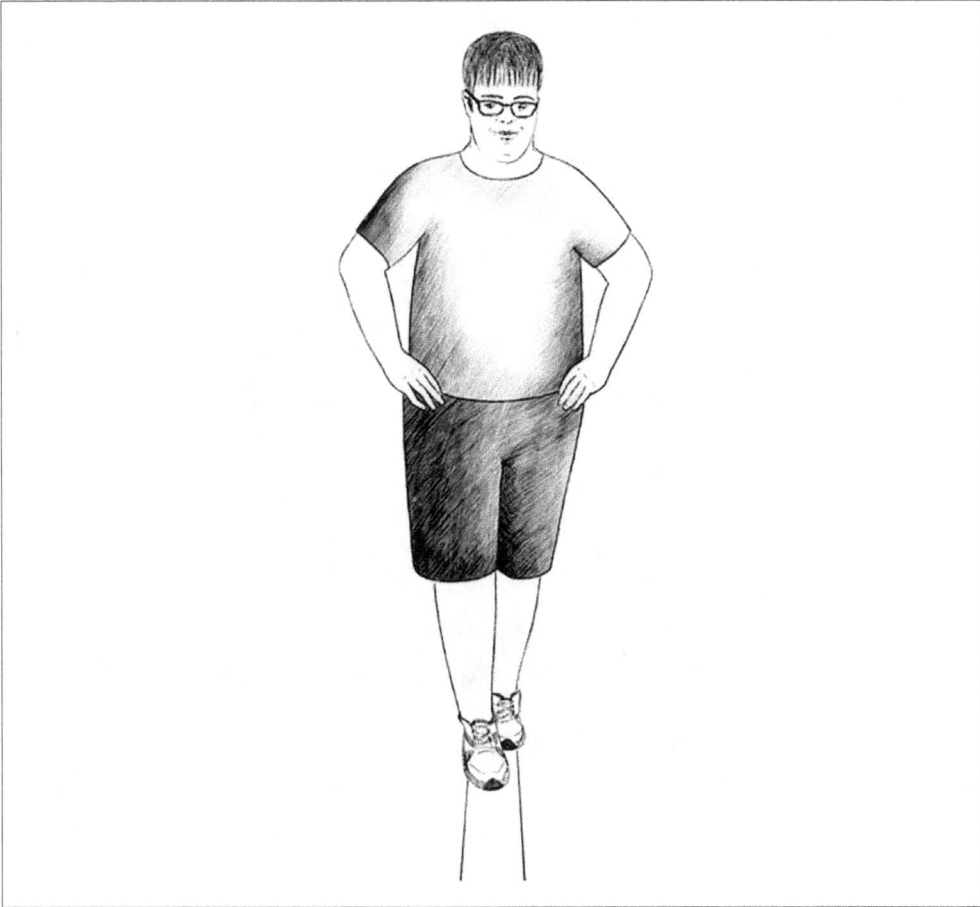

Source: Drawing published with permission from the artist, Luibov Mazanko, c. 2013-2015, Port Elizabeth, South Africa.
FIGURE 4.10: Walking on a balance beam.

Equipment: Cone, folding chair with 43 cm (17 inch) seat height, tape measure and stopwatch.

Procedure: Place the chair against the wall, facing a cone exactly 2.4 m (8 feet) away (measured from the back of the cone to a point at the front edge of the chair). The participant should sit in the middle of the chair, with feet flat on the floor, and the hands on the thighs. One foot may be placed slightly farther than the other and the torso is bent slightly forward. On the signal 'go', the participant gets up from the chair, walks as quickly as possible to the cone, walks around the cone and returns to the chair. No running is allowed (Saunders 2017).

Scoring: After one practice trial, two test trials are administered and the best time is recorded in seconds.

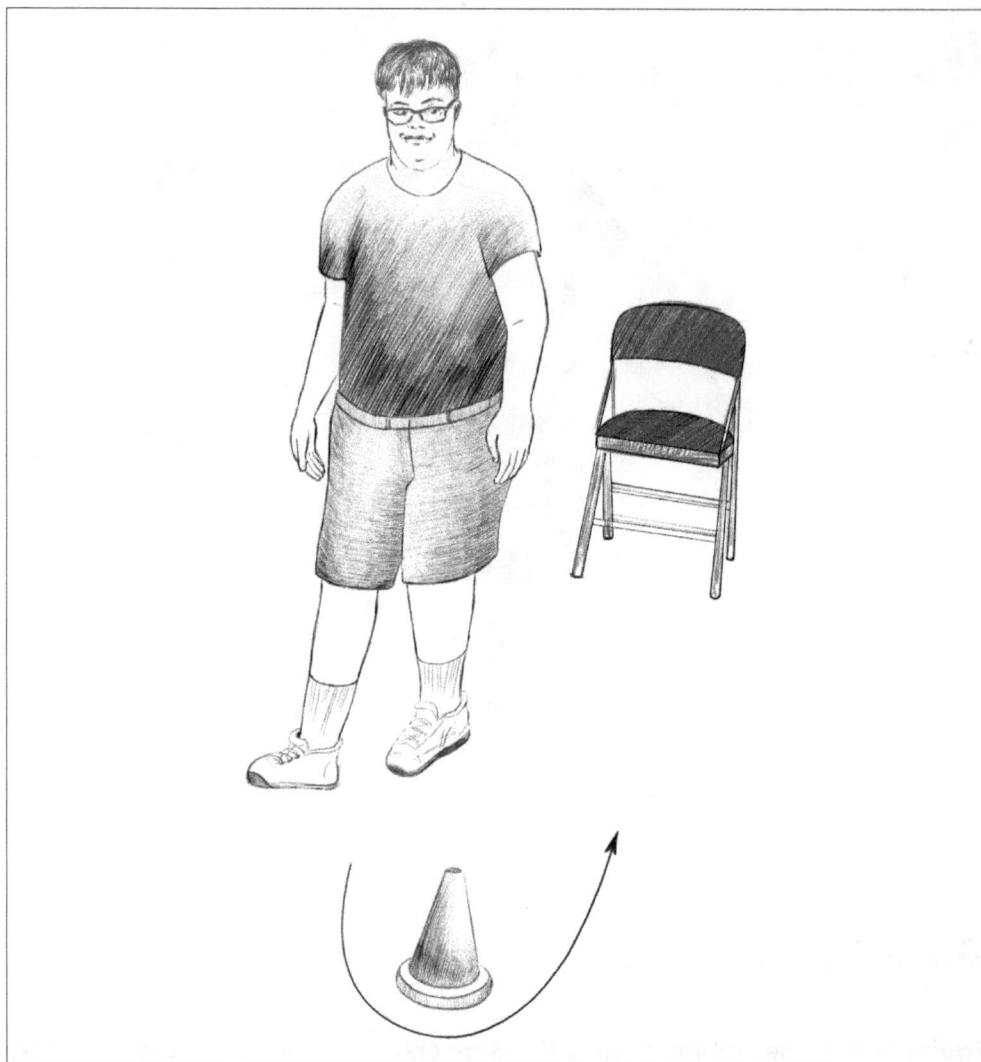

Source: Drawing published with permission from the artist, Luibov Mazanko, *c.* 2013-2015, Port Elizabeth, South Africa.
FIGURE 4.11: 8-foot up-and-go test.

Safety precaution and general instructions: Stand between the cone and the chair in case the participant loses his or her balance. Motivation is key. No running is allowed. When the participant returns to the seated position, his or her back must touch the back of the chair.

☐ Body mass index (height and weight)

Purpose: To assess BMI (see Figure 4.12).

Equipment: Calibrated scale, 150-cm tape measure, masking tape and ruler.

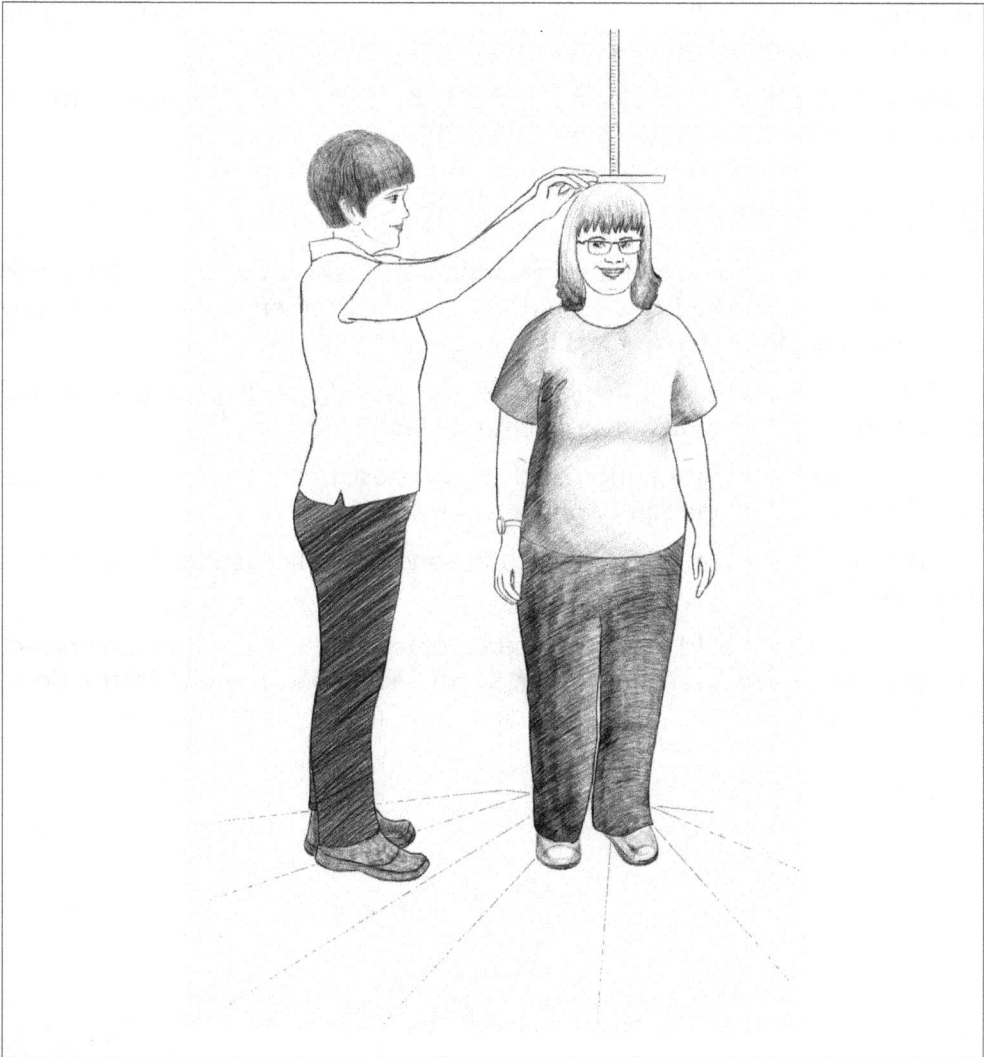

Source: Drawing published with permission from the artist, Luibov Mazanko, c. 2013-2015, Port Elizabeth, South Africa.
FIGURE 4.12: Stature.

Procedure: Participant should only wear his or her shorts and T-shirt or similar lightweight clothing. Ensure the scale is on a level and solid surface (no carpet). Ask the participant to stand in the centre of the scale with his or her weight evenly distributed.

Hold the tape measure vertically against the wall with the zero end at exactly 50 cm from the floor. Have the participant stand with the back, head and feet against the wall. Feet should be together. The tape should be lined up against the wall in line with the centre of the body. The head should be placed in the Frankfurt plane. Place a ruler on top of the participant's head, ensuring that it is parallel to the floor. Record the height in cm and add 50 cm (floor to zero point of measuring tape).

Scoring: Determine the participant's BMI by using the following formula: ($BMI = kg/m^2$).

■ Summary

The FFTB is easy to administer for adults living with DS. If all advice and procedures are followed as outlined in this chapter, there should not be any problems. Testing should not last longer than 1 h per participant.

The chapter provides the purpose, equipment needed, procedure and scoring for each of the 12 functional fitness tests.

Other important information such as pre-test procedures, the warm-up, general information and safety precautions are also provided.

It is emphasised that to ensure accurate and scientific testing, the protocols presented herein should be followed.

The instructor should be well prepared before the testing day with respect to equipment needed, testing order, score sheets and pre-test instructions, and should plan a step-by-step testing procedure for the testing day.

Test results

■ Interpreting test scores

The participant's scores for all 12 functional fitness tests are reported on the score sheet by the research scholar or exercise specialist. An example thereof is presented in Table 5.1 and Table 5.2.

Now that the participant knows his or her test score, the academic scholar or exercise specialist can tailor exercise and other interventions to target identified strengths and weaknesses.

In this example, three points can be highlighted:

1. Firstly, the test scores for all 12 functional fitness tests are recorded under the column 'test scores'. After a period of 2 to 3 months, once the participant has been conditioned to the exercises and other interventions prescribed by the research scholar or exercise specialist, the participant can be re-evaluated. The participant will then compare the test scores obtained during the first assessment with those obtained after 2 to 3 months.
2. Secondly, next to the participant's test score, there is a recorded percentile value. These values are obtained from the norm-referenced tables presented in Chapter 3. For instance, the participant in this example obtained a test

How to cite: Boer, P.-H., 2021, 'Test results', in *Functional fitness for adults living with Down syndrome*, pp. 65–71, AOSIS, Cape Town. https://doi.org/10.4102/aosis.2021.BK252.05

TABLE 5.1: Example of a scorecard with personal information and body mass index.

Personal information	Data
Date of test	**25 November 2020**
Name	**John**
Surname	**Davids**
Gender	**Male**
Age	**28 years**
Physical activity (sessions per week)	**One session per week**
Body mass and height (2 tests)	
Height (cm)	**166**
Body mass (kg)	**80**
BMI (kg/m²)	**29.03**

Source: The information is taken from Chapter 6 (Appendix: Case study – Zane Johnson).

TABLE 5.2: Example of a scorecard with functional fitness test results, percentile norms and minimum standards status.

Tests	Test score	Percentile	Meet minimum requirements
1. Flexibility			
1.1. Chair sit-and-reach test (cm)	16	75	Yes
1.2. Back scratch test (cm)	5	70	Yes
2. Functional ability			
2.1. 8-foot up-and-go (s)	6.6	75	Yes
3. Balance			
3.1. Standing on one leg (s)	10	95	Yes
3.2. Walking on balance beam (n)	6	95	Yes
4. Muscular strength and endurance			
4.1. Modified curl-up (n)	31	55	No
4.2. Trunk lift (cm)	36	80	Yes
4.3. 30-second chair stand (n)	11	20	No
4.4. Handgrip strength (kg)	36.9	85	Yes
4.5. Isometric push-up (s)	70	70	No
5. Aerobic tests			
5.1. 6-minute walk distance test (m)	350	No percentiles available	
5.2. 16-metre PACER (shuttles)	13	20	No

Source: The information is taken from Chapter 6 (Appendix: Case study – Zane Johnson).

score of 11 stands in the 30-second chair stand test. If we proceed to the appropriate table in Chapter 3 (noting that the test is the 30-second chair stand test, participant is male and age category is 24–35), we can see that a score of 11 stands equates to a percentile value of 20%. What does this mean? A percentile value of 20% indicates that 80% of peers (same gender and age category) perform better than he or she did. A percentile value of 70% indicates that only 30% of peers (same gender and age category) perform better than he or she did. In this example, the participant has a poor score for leg strength (30-second chair stand test) and aerobic capacity (6-minute walk distance test) necessitating exercise programs focused on these weaknesses. Even though a good score was reported for handgrip strength (85% percentile indicates that only 15% of peers in the same age and gender category perform better than him), the exercise prescription should still include this type of training to maintain or even improve this parameter of functional fitness. However, the key focus of exercise prescription should be tailored to improve individual weaknesses. It must be remembered that functional fitness is an umbrella term for individual physical parameters of flexibility, balance, muscular strength, aerobic capacity, functional ability and BMI. Strengths in some components, but weaknesses in others, do not guarantee a qualitative, independent and functionally mobile life in later years.

3. Lastly, the third column, 'meet minimum requirement', indicates whether the person met (Yes/No) the minimum requirement for that parameter of functional fitness. The criterion-referenced values are based on the 75th percentile for nine of the 12 functional fitness tests (ch. 3). Two of the exceptions are for both flexibility items where percentile values of 40% are indicative of a minimum requirement because of the very flexible nature of DS individuals. These criterion percentiles have been bolded in Chapter 3 for convenience. At this stage, no percentile table exists for one of the aerobic test items, namely the 6-minute walk distance test. Although these norms are based on the subjective opinion of experts in the field of adapted physical activity, further longitudinal research is needed in order to refine and standardise the norms. As presented in the BPFT, these minimal accepted values are high percentiles (75th percentile) to safeguard against a dependent and functionally impaired life in later years (Winnick & Short 2014:29). Minimal values for a specific age group should be high enough to securely withstand normal age-related declines and to avoid progression to values below those associated with dependence later in life. Also, it must be remembered that the functional fitness of adults living with DS is very low compared to not only the general population but also to those living with ID without DS (ch. 1). Knowing that adults living with DS can increase their functional fitness with large improvements, higher percentile values for criterion-referenced values is logical. Consequently, it is recommended not only to study norm-referenced values but also criterion-referenced standards when prescribing exercise. On the other hand, these criterion-referenced values should not be too high as to offset motivation to attain them. Ultimately, the principle of individuality should not be neglected. When prescribing exercise, it must be remembered that each person will react to exercise interventions differently and thus each individual's factors should be carefully accounted for.

■ Motivation, facilitators and barriers to habitual active lifestyle

The results presented in these score sheets should motivate participants to improve their functional fitness. The use of music, strong social support, positive energy and patience are a few examples of tools that intrinsically motivate adults living with DS. The results of the score sheets should be communicated positively, constructively and carefully in order to avoid demotivating participants. It is critically important for the instructor to convey information in such a way that, regardless of age or score, improvement is always possible. Adults living with DS should not be overwhelmed by the many barriers associated with a habitually active lifestyle, but rather recognise the strengths thereof.

A few studies have examined the many facilitators and barriers of physical activity in DS individuals (Boer 2015:20). Mahy et al. (2010:795) identified selected barriers and facilitators towards a physically active lifestyle in adults living with DS. They stipulated the importance of having a supportive person to enforce the physical activity. Often, the caregivers and support staff housed at ID care centres are inactive themselves and unlikely to provide continuous motivation and to make exercise fun and interesting (Heller, Hsieh & Rimmer 2003:161). Exercise scientists, coaches, as well as physically active volunteers and parents are more likely candidates to support and continuously motivate adults living with DS. Perhaps after an extended period (e.g. 12 months), participants will be intrinsically motivated to initiate exercise sessions without external assistance (Boer 2015:20).

Barriers to a physically active life in adults living with DS include insufficient support from others, not wanting to engage in physical activity, and medical or physiological factors (Boer 2015:20; Mahy et al. 2010:795). Once these barriers have been identified, strategies can be implemented to overcome them. For example, Heller et al. (2003) reported that physical activity should be reinforced by caregivers and accessibility to exercise facilities must be improved. Fortunately, a different study by Heller, Hsieh and Rimmer (2004:175) reported that a combined exercise and health education program can significantly and positively ameliorate perceptions of exercise in adults living with DS. These include an improved self-efficacy, less cognitive-emotional barriers, anticipation of more positive results and improved life satisfaction. Many facilitators contributing to a habitual physically active lifestyle were also identified in individuals living with DS. Exercise should be fun, familiar, routine-based and stimulating (Barr & Shields 2011:1020; Boer 2015:20; Mahy et al. 2010:795). The perceptions and attitudes of caregivers toward the competence of adults living with DS and exercise have also been shown to benefit when physical activity was introduced (Shields et al. 2011:360). Future research addressing the facilitators and barriers of exercise will determine the possibility of an unsupervised habitual, long-term physically active lifestyle in adults living with DS. The 'SMART' described in section 'Goal setting' and FFTB described in section 'Progress and re-evaluation' would also act as additional motivation tools.

◼ Goal setting

The use of goal setting according to the acronym 'SMART' is very helpful:

- S: specific
- M: measurable
- A: authentic
- R: realistic
- T: time.

A goal should be specific, measurable, authentic, realistic and achievable within a specific timeframe.

Referring to the example provided at the beginning of this chapter, the participant obtained a score of 6 stands for the 30-second chair stand test which equated to the 20th percentile of individuals in the same age and gender category. A SMART goal could be: 'I want to improve my leg strength as measured by the 30-second chair stand test from 6 to 9 stands within a period of two months. I want to do this with the help of my exercise specialist as he/she will prescribe a variety of leg strength exercises specifically designed to my needs and abilities.'

This goal is specific (leg strength), measurable (6 to 9 stands), authentic (my goal is suited to my needs and abilities), realistic (achieving this goal within 2 months is possible when structured leg strength training sessions are implemented three times a week) and time bound (within 2 months).

◼ Progress and re-evaluation

Being evaluated on training program and re-evaluated with the FFTB will definitely act as a motivation tool. Knowing that one can improve on existing scores with structured exercise training and goal setting, and bear the advantages thereof, will especially motivate an individual for exercise adherence. Having personnel and peers at the ID care centre question and comment on your functional fitness progress can also help, remind and motivate. It can also be helpful to keep a personal logbook for continued monitoring of exercise and SMART goals. Monitoring of health measures such as blood pressure, resting heart rate, blood glucose, cholesterol, heart rate variability, sleep quality and being free from diseases and conditions may also provide the necessary motivation for continued physical activity.

However, it must be stressed that during the period after re-evaluation, continued exercise is to be maintained so that physical activity becomes habitual. Other intrinsic factors enjoyed at this stage (wellbeing, joy of being active, improved body composition, successful attainment of goals) with continued social support should serve as further and more sustainable reasons to develop a habitually active lifestyle. At this point, however, continued goal setting and monitoring of functional fitness should be maintained. It is recommended that evaluation through the FFTB occurs three times per year. Other methods of physical activity (swimming, cycling, gymnasium, cross fit and pilates) could be included to offer variation.

■ Precautions

The focus of all the information presented in this book should be considered general performance guidelines and not as absolute predictors of functional ability later on in life. This key point is also highlighted in the SFT (Rikli & Jones 2013:94). Further longitudinal research is needed to validate the information presented herein.

However, we do feel that the information presented in this book provides previously unavailable standardised functional fitness tests (aerobic endurance, musculoskeletal functioning, balance, function and BMI) and reference values (norm- and criterion-reference tables).

As stated in the 'Motivation, facilitators and barriers to habitual active lifestyle' section, the principle of individuality should not be forgotten. Each adult living with DS has a unique build (height, weight and body fat distribution), unique clinical or physiological conditions, and unique abilities which could affect person differently than the other. Therefore, the recommended fitness standards may not apply equally to all individuals. For example, the 30-second chair stand test is performed on a chair with a seat height of 43 cm, which in turn could negatively or positively influence a very tall or very short person. As such, it is very important to study each participant as his or her own control by testing him or her every 4 months as to ascertain whether improvement has occurred after some exercise intervention.

Lastly, the tests presented in this book included participants living with DS (non-mosaic type). Adults living with mosaic type DS have better physical and cognitive capabilities and the tests presented herein were not standardised to this group of DS individuals. On the other hand, adults living with severe ID may not be able to perform some of the tests presented in this book. Additionally, the majority of participants on which this book was standardised was Caucasian (95% of all cases), and as such might not generally apply to other cultures. Furthermore, to be included for testing, participants had to possess the necessary cognitive ability to understand testing techniques and procedures. Consequently, individuals living with severe ID were excluded from testing. For example, some adults did not understand the importance of a timed test or could not understand the form or technique of the isometric push-up. Lastly, before test participation, adults living with DS had to submit the adapted physical activity readiness questionnaire (completed by the primary physician). They were excluded if any clinical or physiological conditions contraindicated to physical activity were present. As such, the information presented in this book may not be generalised to those with severe physical and IDs.

■ Summary

This chapter provides important information pertaining to the interpretation of test scores. The interpretation in line with norm- and criterion-referenced scores are also explained. Furthermore, information relating to motivation, goal setting, progression and re-evaluation is also provided.

The norm- and criterion-referenced tables obtained from a nationwide study (371 adults living with DS) are provided in Chapter 3.

Administering the FFTB could act as a helpful motivational tool to inspire adults living with DS to improve their functional fitness. The use of music, social support, accessible and readily available equipment and trainers, as well as the use of logbooks and SMART goals can effectively engage adults living with DS to pursue a habitually active lifestyle.

Exercise recommendations and complete case study for adults living with Down syndrome

◼ Physical activity for adults living with Down syndrome

The ACSM recommends that all adults partake in at least 30 min of moderate physical activity 5 days, if not all days, per week (Pescatello & Riebe 2014). The ACSM also launched a campaign 'Exercise is Medicine ©' which is gaining momentum and popularity amongst all health practitioners worldwide.

Unfortunately, most individuals living with DS live sedentary lifestyles (Boer 2015:31; Esposito et al. 2012:109; Nordstrøm et al. 2013:4395; Shields, Dodd & Abblitt 2009:307). Only 42% of children living with DS performed at least 60 min of moderate to vigorous exercise per day (Shields et al. 2009:307). Another study reported that young children living with DS (3–10 years) did not meet the required vigorous activity per day when compared to their non-

How to cite: Boer, P.-H., 2021, 'Exercise recommendations and complete case study for adults living with Down syndrome', in *Functional fitness for adults living with Down syndrome*, pp. 73–86, AOSIS, Cape Town. https://doi.org/10.4102/aosis.2021.BK252.06

DS peers (Whitt-Glover, O'Neill & Stettler 2006:158). A review article confirmed these findings in children and adolescents living with DS (Pitetti, Baynard & Agiovlasitis 2013:47). Moreover, they illustrated that the amount of physical activity decreased from childhood to adulthood. This may indicate that the root of a habitually sedentary lifestyle is established at a very young age. A study conducted in Norway reported that only 12% of adults living with DS, Prader-Willi syndrome and Williams's syndrome (18–45 years) met the required physical activity levels (Nordstrøm et al. 2013:4395). Furthermore, adults living with DS were the least active of these three groups.

Hopefully, the functional fitness instruments presented in this book along with the norm- and criterion-referenced tables, logbooks, SMART goal setting, strong social support structures with research scholars and conditioning coaches, continued monitoring of progress and re-evaluation, and the many facilitators to physical activity in a DS population presented in Chapter 5 would encourage a habitual physically active lifestyle.

■ Principles of exercise prescription

Exercise prescription should be based on the following five principles (Kenney, Wilmore & Costill 2015):

1. **Principle of individuality –** Not one adult living with DS has the same build, physiology, past training history, past or current injuries, private home or group home, initial functional fitness or genetic material to another adult living with DS. Moreover, all people react differently to the type, duration, volume and intensity of exercise prescription. Some of us prefer indoor activities, others prefer swimming and others enjoy walking in the park. Consequently, no training program should be the same from one person to the other. If the exercise specialist screened each participant (age, gender, previous training, injuries, BMI, resting heart rate and parameters associated with health) with the use of the results obtained from the FFTB, he or she should be able to design an individualised training program.

2. **Principle of specificity –** The training program should be specified to the needs of each participant. Once individual strengths and weaknesses in functional fitness have been identified, the exercise specialist should tailor these specifically for each individual. If poor values for aerobic endurance and leg strength were obtained, these should be focused on during training sessions. As stated previously, strengths in certain parameters should not be neglected and should be maintained or improved.

3. **Principle of reversibility –** If training is decreased or stopped, the physiological adaptations that followed training will be reversed. All exercise programs should consist of a maintenance plan to prevent reversibility. Exercise prescription should be structured in such a way that it would promote a habitual physical active lifestyle.

4. **Principle of periodisation –** The long-term plan of each adult living with DS should be broken into periods. If the long-term plan is based on a year, the year could be divided into quarters to monitor progress through continued re-evaluation with the FFTB. For instance, during the first quarter of the year, the participant would like to improve all weak physical parameters by 20% whereas during the second quarter he or she would like to increase them by another 10%. Perhaps, the exercise specialist recommends more aerobic activities (involving walking) during the first phase and some jogging in the second phase. This principle will be followed to achieve the SMART goals referred to in the latter part of Chapter 5.

5. **Principle of progressive overload –** This principle states that progression should be slow but sustainable over time. Through this principle, injuries, overreaching and symptoms of burn-out will be avoided. Many participants start with an exercise training program over-enthusiastically, and perhaps too quickly, which is not sustainable. As a result, a habitual active lifestyle is not achieved.

■ Lifestyle exercises

When the word 'exercise' is used, many people are immediately discouraged as it refers to something that is structured and mundane. It must be noted that there are studies that report an unhealthy lifestyle even when the participant might engage in 30 min of physical activity every day.

There are many ways that one can be more active just by changing many components in one's everyday life. Each day there are numerous opportunities in which one can be more active if one chooses to do so. A few examples are listed below:

- Walking in town for donations.
- Parents or guardians parking further away from the shop.
- Introducing DS adults to physically active workshops designed for the general population.
- Taking the stairs.
- Engaging in household tasks such as gardening, vacuuming, cleaning and other chores.
- Walking or cycling to work or the shop.
- Joining a hiking club, CrossFit club, pilates club or dancing club.
- Walking along if a family member is playing golf.
- Engaging in physically active vacations (camping, hiking and shopping).
- Lifestyle exercises can also be tailored and individualised to the results obtained from a functional fitness assessment.
- If you use public transport, rather stand than sit.
- Walking to town to buy groceries.

- Go for a walk during your lunch hour at work.
- Stand every 30 min if you are working behind a desk and perform a few basic movements such as squats, lunges, hops or stretches.
- Use more time at home to do physical things rather than watching TV.
- Walk around if you are talking on your mobile phone.

■ Structured exercise

Many studies have been conducted on individuals living with DS and have reported benefits and improvements with structured exercise (Mendonca & Pereira 2009:33; Mendonca, Pereira & Fernhall 2013:353; Shields & Taylor 2010; Tsimaras et al. 2003:1239). Some of these studies included walking on a treadmill (Carmeli et al. 2002:106), aerobic activities such as jogging and cycling (Boer & Moss 2016a:322; Mendonca & Pereira 2009:33), interval training (Boer & Moss 2016a:322), strength training (Shields et al. 2013:4385; Shields & Taylor 2010:187), combined aerobic and strength training (Dodd & Shields 2005:2051; Mendonca et al. 2013:353; Mendonca, Pereira & Fernhall 2011:37; Rimmer et al. 2004:165), balance training (Carmeli et al. 2002:106; Tsimaras & Fotiadou 2004:343), aquatic training (Boer & De Beer 2019:1453) or freestyle swim training (Boer 2020:770). In these studies, many parameters associated with health (BMI, body fat percentage, blood pressure, resting heart rate, etc.), functional ability (everyday living activities), strength (maximal and endurance), fitness (time to exhaustion, VO_2 max) and balance improved significantly.

Aerobic conditioning is important to improve the function of the heart, lungs, blood vessels and muscles. In the FFTB, aerobic conditioning was assessed with the 6-minute walk distance test and the 16-metre PACER test (jogging). Aerobic endurance for adults living with DS can be improved with walking activities (30 min, 3 times per week) using modalities consisting of walking (Carmeli et al. 2002:106), jogging (Boer & Moss 2016a:327; Tsimaras et al. 2003:1239), cycling (Mendonca & Pereira 2009:33), rowing (Varela et al. 2001:135), interval training (Boer & Moss 2016:327), aquatic training (Boer & De Beer 2019:1453) or swim training (Boer 2020:770). It has been reported that leg strength is associated with aerobic ability in DS individuals (Pitetti & Boneh 1995:423). Consequently, concomitant leg strength training could provide the necessary musculature to assist in improvement of aerobic capacity. Studies have shown that aerobic exercise combined with resistance training have also improved the aerobic capacity of these individuals (Lewis & Fragala-Pinkham 2005:30; Mendonca et al. 2011:37, 2013:353; Oviedo et al. 2014:2624; Rimmer et al. 2004:165). It is important to improve the aerobic capacity of adults living with ID or DS as it has been reported that those with the lowest aerobic capacity had the highest body fat percentages (Salaun & Berthouze-Aranda 2012:231). As a result, a well-balanced diet prescribed by a registered dietician may assist with the necessary weight loss and probable improvements in aerobic capacity. Aerobic exercise or combined aerobic and resistance training have been shown to decrease body mass or body fat percentage in individuals living with DS (Boer & Moss 2016a:322; Mendonca & Pereira 2009:33; Ordonez, Rosety & Rosety-Rodriguez 2006:416; Rimmer et al. 2004:165). Aerobic testing should start with light aerobic activities and progress slowly depending on the individual. The principles as highlighted at the start of this chapter should be applied. Aerobic activity should be improved until the participant can exercise comfortably for 30 min, 5 days per week, at a moderate intensity.

The improvement of upper and lower body strength is also important for adults living with DS, as adequate strength is needed for everyday living activities, work and recreational activities, good posture and other tasks such as climbing stairs. Adequate strength levels could also prevent or reduce the probability of future falls, and health-related conditions such as lower back pain, osteoarthritis, low bone mineral density and cardiovascular disease. The importance of adequate strength in adults living with DS is also important as many DS individuals perform physical-rather than cognitive-related work. In addition, improvements in strength assisted these individuals with everyday ADL (Carmeli et al. 2002:106; Cowley et al. 2011:2229; Shields, Taylor & Dodd 2008:1215). Strength training has been performed with individuals living with DS (Cowley et al. 2011:2229; Mendonca et al. 2013:353; Shields et al. 2008:1215; Shields & Taylor 2010:187; Tsimaras & Fotiadou 2004:343). In the study by Mendonca et al. (2013:356), resistance training occurred twice a week and included all major muscle groups of both the lower and upper body. They included single and multiple joint exercises. The circuit of exercises included nine exercises with each exercise being performed twice (shoulder press, chest-press, vertical traction, lower back extension, leg extension, triceps push-down and biceps curl). Participants starting with a resistance training program should ideally perform 8 to 12 repetitions at 70% of 1 repetition maximum. Strength training should be performed with the right technique and the use of an exercise specialist is essential. It is recommended that strength training is performed twice a week for all the major muscle groups (shoulder, chest, bicep, triceps, forearm, upper back, lower back, core, abdominal, quadriceps, hamstrings and gastrocnemius). At least 48 h of recovery is needed between strength training sessions. If or when resistance training equipment is not available, participants living with DS can use their own body weight (e.g. push-ups, dips, pull-ups, standing squats and lunges, and wall sits) or natural obstacles such as staircases can be used.

Improving flexibility is also an important component of functional fitness. Although most adults living with DS have more-than-optimal upper and lower body flexibility (Boer 2010:78), the maintenance of adequate flexibility remains crucial. Good posture, the prevention of injuries and everyday living activities such as dressing, pulling a seatbelt over your shoulder and brushing your teeth necessitate a good range of motion around a joint. Stretching exercises should be avoided by adults with DS, unless an adapted exercise specialist is present. Because of the hyper-mobility, ligamentous laxity and poor muscle tone of adults living with DS, injuries could occur. If exercise professional is present, stretching exercises should be performed for all major muscle and joint areas such as the ankle, knee, hip, back, trunk, neck and shoulder. Static stretching should be performed during the cool-down period when the participant slowly stretches the muscle into the end position and holds it for 10 s to 30 s. Dynamic stretching exercises should be performed during the warm-up with movement of the joint occurring through the full range of motion (e.g. swinging the legs). Correct technique is important, with no bouncing and jerking movements. No pain should be felt during any stretching exercises.

Lastly, balance exercises are also important for adults living with DS. The ability to balance optimally requires input from many sources such as musculoskeletal, central nervous system, coordination, visual and somatosensory. Static and dynamic balance is required for many activities such as walking, climbing stairs, hiking and showering. Having good balance could possibly prevent future falls, especially in old age. Static balance can be improved with activities such as standing on one leg (with eyes open or with eyes closed), lunging on one leg, squatting on one leg and reaching to an object whilst standing on one leg. Dynamic balance can be improved with agility ladders or hurdles, walking on a balance beam, playing tennis or bowls and dancing. Balance ability has improved significantly in previous studies conducted on individuals living with DS with suitable intervention strategies (Carmeli et al. 2002:106; Lewis & Fragala-Pinkham 2005:30; Tsimaras & Fotiadou 2004:343).

A few examples of exercises to improve strength, flexibility and balance are provided by Rikli and Jones (2013:114). The studies using the exercises provided in this chapter may assist with training examples specific to a population of individuals living with DS. The 'Complete case study' section provides an example of a complete case study by using the FFTB as described in this book.

■ Complete case study: An example of how to use the information presented in this book

A participant visited the adapted physical activity specialist, wanting to be assessed with the FFTB.

It is suggested that the following steps are followed as outlined in Appendix H:

1. The adapted physical activity specialist advises the participant to visit his primary health care practitioner with the adapted physical activity

readiness questionnaire (app. G) to verify whether he or she is ready to perform physical activity. The following page provides an example of the successful completion of this form.

2. The adapted physical activity specialist should carefully study the contents presented in this book. Especially, the methodology section presented in Chapter 4 should be studied in detail.

3. The adapted physical activity specialist provides the participant and his or her parent or guardian with the consent form, as well as a short verbal and physical description and demonstration of all 12 functional fitness tests (app. A). The activity specialist also provides the participant with the form of important information pertaining to 24 h before the test (app. B). After a minimum of 5 days has elapsed, the informed consent form is collected. The activity specialist and the participant's parent or guardian identify an appropriate date for exercise testing to commence at 09:00 in the morning.

4. The adapted physical activity specialist obtains the page outlining equipment needed (app. C), order of tests and stations (app. D) and the participant score sheet (app. E).

5. The adapted physical activity specialist sets up the test venue with equipment as stipulated in Appendix D and Appendix E.

6. The adapted physical activity exercise specialist instructs the participant to complete all 14 tests (including height and weight). The contents of Chapter 4 and the information provided in Appendix D provide clear guidelines. The 6-minute walk distance test is always performed last. The 16-metre shuttle run test is always performed on the following day. Appendix E is completed to capture the test information and performance of the adult living with DS.

7. The participant's test score is recorded and compared with the normative tables found in Chapter 3. Whether the participant's test score reaches minimal acceptable standards should also be recorded. See bolded rows in the various tables depicted in Chapter 3. The form from Appendix F is used for completion of this step.

8. The adapted physical activity exercise specialist provides the participant with exercises to maintain existing strengths and improve weaknesses (ch. 6). Importantly, it is best to compare Zane's own functional fitness scores before a period of exercise intervention to his scores after a period of exercise intervention. However, comparing his scores to norm- and criterion-referenced scores provides additional information which is useful (ch. 3). The BMI of Zane places him in the obese category (> 30). Although an exercise intervention is needed, BMI should be interpreted cautiously in this population who are known to have short stature and thus higher BMI values. If it is possible, and his parents or guardian has the financial means, further analyses of percentage body fat, waist and hip circumference would provide more specific information pertaining to his anthropometry. Percentage body fat can be determined by skinfold measurements, bio-electrical impedance analysis or even more

advanced techniques. The FFTB instrument as provided in this book provides field-based tests that are accessible to most individuals and as a consequence, BMI is used as with other well-known field-based instruments (Hilgenkamp, Van Wijck & Evenhuis 2012; Rikli & Jones 2013; Winnick & Short 2014). It must be noted that ultimately a prediction formula is used to determine percentage body fat when using any technique and that there will always be a margin of error with these sophisticated techniques. Nevertheless, an exercise intervention targeting a reduction in body mass is important for Zane.

Zane's strengths are his upper and lower body flexibility. Again, as advised, flexibility training should be performed by a trained specialist as adults living with DS have hypermobile joints and suffer from ligamentous laxity. Zane could easily injure himself if the stretching movements are not performed correctly. Flexibility training should be performed under the supervision of a trained exercise professional.

Zane does not meet the minimum requirements for the rest of the functional fitness test items. He is placed at the 50th percentile for the modified curl-up (abdominal strength) and handgrip strength. Scores at the 50th percentile indicate that 50% of adult men living with DS, who are in the age category of 18–25, perform better than him in this test. The rest of his scores appear below the 50th percentile. An exercise program should be prescribed for Zane so that he can improve on all functional fitness parameters. The principles of exercise prescription as presented in Chapter 6 should be adhered to.

Depending on his financial means and access to equipment and facilities, a specific program could be developed for him. For example, if he has access to a gymnasium, a park, a swimming pool, a dance club, a walking club or a sporting club, specific activities could be designed for him. If not, there are a myriad of activities that can be performed at home. The adapted physical activity specialist could help design such a training program. Exercise programs consisting of combined aerobic and resistance type activities have been significant to improve aerobic capacity, body mass, body composition and muscular strength for adults living with DS (González-Agüero et al. 2011:2383; Mendonca, Pereira & Fernhall 2011:37, 2013:356; Rimmer et al. 2004:165) The exercise intervention should be 30 min to 60 min in length and performed three times a week. An example of a possible start to an exercise program performed at home is provided in Table A-1. Please note that this is an example, as the program could be more varied and there are many more exercises that could be considered. No equipment is needed for this exercise program. A 10-s to 30-s break between repetitions and a 1 min break between activities should be provided.

Music should be played during these activities as most adults living with DS are motivated and inspired by their favourite music. Constant motivation and praise should be provided during these activities. Preferably a person close to Zane such as a family member or friend should perform these activities with him to provide further motivation. Progress reports, weekly exercises and charts should be stuck to his wall to provide more inspiration and feelings of accomplishment. Additional facilitators and barriers to physical activity are provided in Chapter 5. This may also help Zane to overcome the many barriers that individuals living with DS face.

If aerobic, water aerobic, swimming, hiking and dancing activities could be incorporated for adults living with DS, it will help with motivation and program diversity (Boer 2020:770; Boer & De Beer 2019:1453; Reinders, Bryden & Fletcher 2015:291). A study by Boer and Moss (2016a:322) and Boer et al. (2014:221) have also shown that interval training was more significant than traditional continuous aerobic training in improving many parameters of functional fitness for adults living with DS and those living with ID. As a consequence, it would be advised to include high intensity intermittent activities (short or longer intervals) combined with low intensity exercise or rest. An example would be 30 s of high intensity running or uphill walking combined with 90 s of rest. Ten sets of these are performed. If it is possible, interval training is easily performed on a treadmill or bicycle ergometer. Most adults living with DS cannot tolerate high speeds on the treadmill and as a consequence it is best to set the incline to 6%–10% and perform 30 s of uphill walking, interspersed with 90 s of rest.

9. The participant should be re-assessed after a period of 3 months to monitor progress of the exercise intervention. This re-assessment is crucial to determine whether the exercise program has been successful. The principle of individuality (ch. 6) is important in this regard as each individual acts as his or her own control. At this stage, the exercise protocol can be adapted according to the magnitude of improvements for each component of functional fitness.

10. A lifelong habitual physical active lifestyle is important for adults living with DS. Physical activity should become part of their normal daily routine.

◼ Summary

This chapter provided an overview of the exercise recommendations and lifestyle activities for adults living with DS. It also provided a complete case study.

■ Appendix: Case study – Zane Johnson

BOX 6A-1: Adapted physical activity readiness questionnaire – Zane Johnson.

Regular physical activity is fun and healthy and more people should increase their physical activity every day. Being more physically active is very safe for MOST people.

Please read the questions carefully and answer each one honestly. If you have any concerns about your health status, you should check with your doctor before becoming more physically active.

Question		Yes	No
1	Has your doctor ever said that you have a heart condition OR high blood pressure?		x
2	Do you feel pain in your chest at rest, during your daily activities of living, OR when you do physical activity?		x
3	Do you lose balance because of dizziness OR have you lost consciousness (fainted) in the last 12 months?		x
4	Have you ever been diagnosed by a health professional as having any of the following (Check all that apply)?		

	Heart trouble		Arthritis		Back problems
	High blood pressure		Chronic asthma		Foot problems
	High cholesterol		Emphysema		Allergies
	Diabetes		Bronchitis		Trouble hearing

Question			Yes	No
5	Are you currently taking any medication for any of the conditions listed above?	*Please describe:*		x
6	Do you have a bone or joint problem that could be made worse by becoming more physically active? (if you had a joint problem in the past, e.g. knee, ankle and shoulder, please answer NO to this question).			x
7	Has your Doctor, Nurse Practitioner (or health provider) ever said that you should only do medically supervised physical activity?			x

Acknowledgement		
8	I have read and understood the above health questions and directions regarding my participation in the Fit, Fun & Fully Alive! Group Fitness Classes.	Your Initials __ZJ_____

Disclaimer

IF YOU ANSWERED YES to one or more of the questions above, you should consult your doctor or health provider first before becoming more physically active. Talk with your doctor about the kinds of activities you wish to participate in and follow his or her advice.

IF YOU ANSWERED NO to all the questions above, you can be reasonably sure that you can start becoming more physically active.
• Begin slowly and build up gradually. Delay becoming more active if you are not feeling well because of a temporary illness such as a cold or a fever wait until you feel better.
• If your health changes so that you would answer YES to any of the PAR-Q questions, ask for advice from your health professional and let your Fitness Instructor know.

BOX 6A-2: Participant raw scorecard – Zane Johnson.

Personal information				
Name:	Zane	**Surname:**		Johnson
Gender:	Male	**Age:**		25 years
Level of education:	Special school	**Type of DS:**		Trisomy 21
Living arrangement:	Care centre	**Physical activity:**		2/week

Body mass and height (two tests)				
Height:	160	cm	**Body mass:**	79 kg

Functional fitness (12 tests)

Aerobic tests (two tests)

6-minute walk distance	10, 25 (50 yard per lap)	laps	468.6 (512, 5 yards)	metres
16-metre PACER	2, 4	level	11	shuttles

Flexibility (2 tests)

Chair sit-and-reach test	Left leg:	Trial 1:	8	cm	Trial 2:	9	cm
	Right leg:	Trial 1:	10	cm	Trial 2:	11	cm
Back scratch test	Left shoulder:	Trial 1:	4	cm	Trial 2:	2	cm
	Right shoulder:	Trial 1:	6	cm	Trial 2:	7	cm

Muscular strength and endurance (five tests)

Handgrip strength	Left hand	Trial 1:	20	kg	Trial 2: 25	kg	Trial 3: 21	kg
	Right hand	Trial 1:	30	kg	Trial 2: 31	kg	Trial 3: 27	kg
Isometric push-up		Trial 1:	30	sec				
Trunk lift		Trial 1:	23	cm	Trial 2:	26	cm	
Modified curl-up		Trial 1:	16	amount				
30-second chair stand test		Trial 1:	11	amount	Trial 2:	11	amount	

Balance (two tests)

Standing on one leg	Left leg	Trial 1:	7	sec	Trial 2:	6	sec
	Right leg	Trial 1:	4	sec	Trial 2:	2	sec
Walking on the balance beam		Trial 1:	4	steps	Trial 2:	3	steps

Functional Test

8-foot up-and-go test	Trial 1:	5.21	sec	Trial 2:	5.35	sec

BOX 6A-3: Raw scorecard and percentile norms – Zane Johnson.

Personal information					
Name	Zane		Surname	Johnson	
Gender	Male		Age	25 years	
Physical activity (sessions per week)	2		Date of test	20 Jan 2020	
Body mass and height					
Height (cm)	160 cm (1.60 m)	Body mass (kg)	79 kg	BMI (kg/m²)	79 kg / ([1.6]2) = 30.86

Functional fitness tests				
Test		Test score	Percentile	Meet minimum requirements
1. Flexibility	1.1. Chair sit-and-reach test (n) (RS)	11	60	Yes
	1.2. Back scratch test (cm) (RS)	7	80	Yes
2. Functional ability	2.1. 8-foot up-and-go (s)	5.21	40	No
3. Balance	3.1. Standing on one leg (s) (RS)	7	40	No
	3.2. Walking on balance beam (steps)	4	35	No
4. Muscular strength and endurance	4.1. Modified curl-up (n)	16	50	No
	4.2. Trunk lift (cm)	25	30	No
	4.3. 30-second chair stand test (n)	11	20	No
	4.4. Handgrip strength (kg) (RS)	31	50	No
	4.5. Isometric push-up (s)	30	25	No
5. Aerobic tests	5.1. 6-minute walk distance test (m)	469	n/a	n/a
	5.2. 16-metre PACER (shuttles)	11	15	No

Note: RS, right-hand side.

BOX 6A-4: An example of a possible start to a training program adapted to the needs of Zane

Training program		
Week 1		
Monday	Wednesday	Friday
• 20 min of walking	• 25 min of walking	• 20 min of walking
• 1x [10 squats, 10 walking lunges]	• 1x [8x trunk lifts]	• 5x [vertical jump]
• 1x [10-s plank on elbows]	• 1x [10-s side plank on elbow, both sides]	• 1x [10-s plank on elbows, both sides]
• 1x [20-s isometric push-up]	• 1-min of running on the spot	• 1x [20-s isometric push-up]
• 1x [10 crunches]	• 2x [10x sit-ups]	• 1x [10 bicycle crunches]
• 1x [15 pillow slams]	• 2x [5x push-up or adapted push-up]	• 1x [20 pillow slams]
• 1x [10 shoulder press using tinned food in each hand]	• 1x [10-s side plank on elbow, both sides]	• 1x [10-s wall sit]
• 1x [15 calf raises]	• 2x [10x frog jumps]	• 5x [standing long jump]
• 2x [standing on one leg for as long as possible for each leg]	• 1x [walking 10-m in semi-squatted position]	• 1x [20 walking lunges]
• 1x [8 x bicep curls using tinned food in each hand]	• 2x [8x flies using tinned food in each hand]	• 1x [10 hand walk-ins from standing to near prone position]
• 1x [8 x tricep dips using a chair]	• 2x [8x lie down and stand-up]	• 1x [10x overhead tin claps]
• 1x [10-m bear walk]	• 2x [25-m sprints]	• 1x [10x calf raises]
Week 2		
Monday	Wednesday	Friday
• 15 min of walking	• 20 min of walking (last 5 min is slow jogging)	• 10x (30-s uphill moderate intensity walking followed by 90 s of rest)
• 5x [20-m sprints]		
• 1x [15 squats, 10 walking lunges]	• 1x [10x trunk lifts]	• 6x [vertical jump]
• 1x [15-s plank on elbows]	• 1x [10-s side plank on elbow, both sides]	• 2x [10-s plank on elbows]
• 1x [20-s isometric push-up]	• 1-min of running on the spot	• 1x [20-s isometric push-up]
• 1x [15 crunches]	• 2x [10x sit-ups]	• 1x [12 bicycle crunches]
• 1x [20 pillow slams]	• 2x [5x push-up or ladies push-up]	• 1x [20 pillow slams]
• 1x [10 shoulder press using tinned food in each hand]	• 1x [10-s side plank on elbow, both sides]	• 1x [12-s wall sit]
• 1x [20 calf raises]	• 2x [12 frog jumps]	• 5x [standing long jump]
• 2x [standing on one leg for as long as possible for each leg]	• 1x [walking 10-m in semi-squatted position]	• 1x [20 walking lunges]
• x [10x bicep curls using tinned food in each hand]	• 2x [8x flies using tinned food in each hand]	• 1x [10 hand walk-ins from standing to near prone position]
• 1x [8x tricep dips using a chair]	• 3x [8x lie down and stand-up]	• 1x [12x overhead tin claps]
• 1x [10-m bear walk]	• 2x [30-m sprints]	• 1x [12x calf raises]

BOX 6A-4 continues on the next page→

BOX 6A-4 (Continues...): An example of a possible start to a training program adapted to the needs of Zane

Week 3		
Monday	Wednesday	Friday
• 20 min of walking (first and last 5 min = slow jogging)	• 25 min of walking	• 10x (30-s uphill moderate intensity walking followed by 90 s of rest)
• 2x [10 squats, 10 walking lunges]	• 1x [12x trunk lifts]	• 5x [vertical jump]
• 2x [10-s plank on elbows]	• 1x [10-s side plank on elbow, both sides]	• 1x [10-s plank on elbows, both sides]
• 2x [20-s isometric push-up]	• 1-min of running on the spot	• 2x [20-s isometric push-up]
• 2x [10 crunches]	• 2x [10x sit-ups]	• 1x [15 bicycle crunches]
• 2x [15 pillow slams]	• 2x [5x push-up or ladies push-up]	• 2x [20 pillow slams]
• 2x [10 shoulder press using tinned food in each hand]	• 1x [10-s side plank on elbow, both sides]	• 1x [10-s wall sit]
• 2x [15 calf raises]	• 2x [10 frog jumps]	• 5x [standing long jump]
• 2x [standing on one leg for as long as possible for each leg]	• 1x [walking 10-m in semi-squatted position]	• 2x [20 walking lunges]
• 2x [8x bicep curls using tinned food in each hand]	• 2x [8x flies using tinned food in each hand]	• 2x [10 hand walk-ins from standing to near prone position]
• 2x [8x tricep dips using a chair]	• 1x [8x lie down and stand-up]	• 2x [10x overhead tin claps]
• 1x [10-m bear walk]	• 4x [20-m sprints]	• 2x [10x calf raises]

APPENDICES

Appendix A: Informed consent and assumption of liability

FUNCTIONAL FITNESS TESTING IN ADULTS WITH DOWN SYNDROME	
Written in SIMPLER language for the research participant and his or her guardian.	
1	**Purpose of the assessment**
You are invited to an assessment to evaluate your functional fitness. If you decide that you want to be evaluated, this is what will happen. An adapted physical activity specialist will come to the place where you work or stay and he or she will perform 14 tests on you and your friends. You will be visited on four occasions. Information and demonstration sessions will be conducted on the first two visits. Testing will happen over the next two visits.	
2	**Procedure**
You will be visited on four occasions. On first arrival, consent forms and the adapted physical activity readiness questionnaire (aPARQ) will be handed out (app. G). Your doctor needs to complete the aPARQ form and confirm that you may participate in physical activity. All 14 tests and procedures will be explained and demonstrated so that you have an idea of what to expect. This session will last 30 min.	
On the second visit, consent forms and the aPARQ will be collected from those wishing to participate. Personal information regarding your year of birth, age, sex, marital status and employment status, level of education and type of work will be collected. We will then proceed to measure body mass and body length measurements. Subsequently, you will be familiarised with the other 12 physical fitness tests (balance, muscular strength and endurance, functional and endurance test items). All of these tests have been adapted to those with intellectual disability or elderly in the general population. Also, all of these tests have been conducted previously to 371 adults with Down syndrome with no complications. All tests were shown to be reliable in adults with Down syndrome. In fact, all of the participants enjoyed the testing and wanted to know they will be re-tested. Lastly, a document will be handed out with information regarding the 24 h before final testing. This session will last 2 h.	
On the third visit, the participant will be tested on 11 functional fitness tests. Body mass and height had already been tested on the second visit. This session will last 2 to 3 h.	
On the fourth visit (next day), the participant will complete the last aerobic test item which should last 20 to 25 min. In all, 14 tests will be administered.	
3	**Can anything bad happen to me?**
In the one test, you will get tired and sweat a bit, your heart will beat fast and you will breathe rapidly. People will be there to help you. You will not be pushed beyond a point of overexertion and you may stop any test at any time.	
4	**Can anything good happen to me?**
This study will show you that exercise is healthy and fun and we hope to learn something that will help you. The exercise specialist will give you feedback on your results and exercises that you can do to improve on your current functional fitness ability.	
5	**Do I have choices?**
You or your guardian can choose not to be in assessment of functional fitness. You may withdraw at any time you please. You may withdraw even once you have started with the assessment.	

Appendix A continues on the next page →

6	Will anyone know I did this assessment?

The exercise specialist would not tell anyone that you were assessed. It remains your choice what the exercise specialist should do with your results. The results of your assessment will not be used for research purposes as to identify you.

7	What happens if I feel anxious or scared?

If you fall or feel unwell, the exercise specialist will be there to help and comfort you and help you get better. If you feel, that your parent or guardian or a nurse or doctor or someone from the care centre should be there during assessment, it is totally permissible and advised. If you feel shy, a professional worker or parent from the place where you stay will be there to help and comfort you. Similarly, if you feel anxious or scared a professional worker or your parent from the place where you stay will be there to help and comfort you.

8	What if I do not want to do this?

You do not have to be in functional fitness assessment. It is up to you. If you say yes now, but you change your mind later, that is okay too. All you have to do is tell us. If you have any more questions, please ask your parent or guardian or the exercise specialist. If you want to be in this study, please sign or print your name.

9	Questions?

You are welcome to ask any questions before you decide to give consent. You can call the exercise specialist at any time for additional questions. Your parent or guardian also has to sign this form and can direct any questions to the exercise specialist.

10	Feedback of findings

The findings of your evaluation will be shared with you in a feedback session to be scheduled after assessment. The exercise specialist will provide information as how you can improve your functional assessment. If you agree, re-assessment should be performed after approximately 3 months of training.

CONSENT FORM

Participation in this research is voluntary (it is your and your parents or guardians choice whether you want to be evaluated).

You are free to decline to take part in this study, or to withdraw at any point even after you have signed the form to give consent, without any consequences.

Should you be willing to participate, you are requested to complete and sign below:

I, _____ hereby voluntarily consent to participate in the above-mentioned assessment. I am not coerced (forced) in any way to participate and I understand that I can withdraw at any time should I feel uncomfortable during the study. I also understand that my name will not be disclosed (revealed) to anybody who is not part of the assessment and that the information will be kept confidential (private) and not linked to my name at any stage. I also understand what I might benefit from participation as well as what might be the possible risks and should I need further information, someone will be available to assist me. My primary physician has agreed for me to participate in physical activity.

_____ Date	_____ Signature of the participant
_____ Date	_____ Signature of the parent or guardian

Appendix B: Participant instructions before assessment

FUNCTIONAL FITNESS INSTRUCTIONS BEFORE ASSESSEMENT	
Please read through the following reminders before the day of assessment	
Name and Surname	
Date and time of assessment:	
Place of assessment:	
1	No coffee or alcohol should be consumed before 24 h of testing.
2	No excessive exercise should be performed 24 h prior to testing.
3	Remember to submit your completed and signed informed consent and adapted physical activity readiness questionnaire, 3 days before exercise testing (Appendixes A and G).
4	Eat a light meal 1 or 2 h before assessment.
5	Inform the exercise specialist of any medical conditions or medications that could affect your performance.
6	You should be familiarised with all 14 tests before the day of assessment. This should have been done during the second visit (Appendix A). Familiarisation sessions will help with pacing strategies on testing day.

Appendix C: Equipment needed

FUNCTIONAL FITNESS EQUIPMENT NEEDED	
Test Items	**Equipment**
General	Pen, recording sheet, clipboard, stopwatch, cones, 50 cm steel ruler and measuring table (20 m and 5 m)
Body mass and height	Calibrated electronic scale, 150-cm tape measure, prestic and steel ruler
Standing on one leg	Stopwatch
Walking on balance beam	Balance beam (3.05 m in length and 10.16 cm wide)
Back scratch	50-cm steel ruler
Sit-and-reach	50-cm steel ruler and 43-cm folding chair
Chair stands (cm)	Stopwatch and 43-cm folding chair
Isometric push-up	Gymnasium mat and stopwatch
Handgrip strength	Handgrip strength dynamometer and 43-cm folding chair
Modified curl-up	Gymnasium mat
Trunk lift	Gymnasium mat and 50-cm steel ruler
8-foot get-up-and-go	Stopwatch, 43-cm folding chair, 5-m tape measure and cone
6-minute walk distance	Stopwatch and eight cones
Bleep shuttles	CD player, 4 cones, 20-m tape measure and bleep test CD

Appendix D: Order of testing and station signs

ORDER OF TESTING AND STATION SIGNS	
A 5-minute break should be provided between all tests.	

Order	Tests
1	Body mass (pre-assessment day)
2	Height (pre-assessment day)
3	Chair sit-and-reach test
4	Back scratch test
5	8-foot get-up-and-go
6	Standing on one leg
7	Walking on the balance beam
8	Modified curl-up
9	Trunk lift
10	30-second chair stand test
11	Handgrip strength
12	Isometric push-up
13	6-minute walk distance test
14	16-metre PACER test (next day)

Appendix D continues on the next page →

TESTING AND STATION SIGNS	
Test 1 and 2	**Body mass and height to calculate body mass index**
Purpose	To assess BMI.
Equipment	Calibrated scale, 150-cm tape measure, masking tape and 50-cm steel ruler.
Procedure	Participant should only wear his or her shorts and T-shirt. Ensure the scale is on a level and solid surface (no carpet). Ask the participant to stand in the centre of the scale with weight evenly distributed. Place the tape measure vertically up the wall with the zero end at exactly 50 cm from the floor. Have the participant stand with the back, head and feet against the wall. Feet should be together. The tape should be lined up against the middle of the head. The head should be placed in the Frankfurt plane. Place a ruler on top of the participants head ensuring that it is parallel to the floor. Record the height in cm and add 50 cm (floor to zero point of measuring tape). *Source*: Drawing published with permission from the artist, Luibov Mazanko, *c.* 2013-2015, Port Elizabeth, South Africa.
Scoring	Determine the participants' BMI with the following formula (BMI = kg/m²).
Safety precautions and general instructions	-

Appendix D continues on the next page →

Test 3	Chair sit-and-reach test
Purpose	To assess lower body flexibility.
Equipment	Folding chair with a seat height of 43 cm (17 inches) will have legs that angle forward to prevent tipping. A steel ruler of at least 50 cm. Chair is placed against the wall.
Procedure	This test is performed twice, first with the one leg and then the other. Two trials on each leg are administered. The leg is extended straight out in front of the hip, with the heel on the floor and the ankle flexed at 90° (the other leg is bent off to the side with the foot flat on the floor). With the hands overlapped and the middle fingers even and on the steel ruler, the participant reached as far as possible to the toes. The maximum reach height must be held for at least 2 s. The same procedure is followed with the other leg. The instructor places one hand with the steel ruler on the participants knee to ensure that there is no knee bend and the other hand on the participants toe also holding the steel ruler. *Source*: Drawing published with permission from the artist, Luibov Mazanko, c. 2013-2015, Port Elizabeth, South Africa.
Scoring	Two practice trials are allowed and then two test trials on each leg. If the tip of the middle finger did not touch the toe, the distance short of the middle toe was measured and recorded as a negative score whilst a middle finger reached beyond the toes, the distance of overlap was measured and recorded as a positive score. Safety and general instructions: Place the chair against the wall. The participant should exhale as he/she stretches. No bouncing movements are allowed. Do not administer the test to participants with knee or hip injuries or that experience pain. The tested leg must remain extended.
Safety and general instructions	Place the chair against the wall. The participant should exhale as he/she stretches. No bouncing movements are allowed. Do not administer the test to participants with knee or hip injuries or that experience pain. The tested leg must remain extended.

Test 4	Back scratch test
Purpose	To assess upper body (shoulder) flexibility.
Equipment	50 cm steel ruler.
Procedure	Participants attempt to touch the fingertips of their two hands behind their back. The participant reaches with his or her right hand in external rotation over the right shoulder between the scapulae, whilst the left elbow is bent and internally rotated and reached upwards from the waist. Direct the participant's middle fingers to each other without helping the stretch. The test is performed on the left and right sides. In both tests, two practice trials are permissible. Two test trials are performed and the best score is noted. The maximum stretch should be held for at least 2 s. *Source*: Drawing published with permission from the artist, Luibov Mazanko, *c.* 2013–2015, Port Elizabeth, South Africa.
Scoring	If the middle fingers of the two hands did not touch, the distance was measured and recorded as a negative score. If the middle fingers overlapped, the distance of overlap was recorded as a positive score.
Safety and general instructions	Stop the test if the participant experiences pain. The participant should exhale as he/she stretches. No bouncing movements are allowed.

Appendix D continues on the next page →

Test 5	8-foot up-and-go test
Purpose	To assess functional ability.
Equipment	Cone, folding chair with 43 cm (17 inch) seat height, tape measure and stopwatch.
Procedure	Place the chair against the wall, facing a cone exactly 2.4 m (8 feet) away (measured from the back of the cone to a point at the front edge of the chair). The participant should sit in the middle of the chair, and feet flat on the floor, with the hands on the thighs. One foot may be slightly ahead of the other and the torso bent slightly forward. On the signal 'go', the participant gets up from the chair, walks as quickly as possible to the cone, walks around the cone and returns to the chair. No running is allowed.
Scoring	After one practice trial, two test trials are administered and the best time is recorded in seconds.

Source: Drawing published with permission from the artist, Luibov Mazanko, c. 2013-2015, Port Elizabeth, South Africa.

Safety and general instructions	Stand between the cone and the chair, so that if the participant loses his or her balance, the instructor is there to help. Motivation is key. No running is allowed. When the participant returns to the seated position his or her back must touch the back of the chair.

Appendix D continues on the next page →

Test 6	Standing on one leg (stalk stand)
Purpose	To assess static balance (see Figure A-5).
Equipment	Stopwatch.
Procedure	This test assesses how long participants can stand on one leg for as long as they can up to a maximum of 10 s. No shoes are allowed. The participant looks straight ahead with their hands on their hips. The knee of the free leg is bent so the lower leg is parallel to the floor. The knee or lower part of the bent leg may not touch the standing leg. The test is performed with both legs and the best score of each leg is noted as static balance performance. Two practice trials and two test trials are administered. The best score is noted. *Source*: Drawing published with permission from the artist, Luibov Mazanko, *c.* 2013–2015, Port Elizabeth, South Africa.
Scoring	The test is terminated once the hands move off the hips and if too much body sway occurs.
Safety precautions and general instructions	Stop the test if the participant experiences pain. Stand next to the participant in case he or she loses balance.

Appendix D continues on the next page →

Test 7	7 Walking on the balance beam
Purpose	To assess dynamic balance (see Figure A-6).
Equipment	Balance beam (3.05 m by 10.16 cm).
Procedure	The participants is instructed to walk with a normal stride, with hands on the hips on the balance beam. The number of consecutive steps completed on the balance beam, up to a maximum of six steps, is recorded. Two practice trials and two test trials are administered. The best score is noted. *Source*: Drawing published with permission from the artist, Luibov Mazanko, *c.* 2013–2015, Port Elizabeth, South Africa.
Scoring	Amount of steps (maximum score is 6).
Safety precautions and general instructions	Walk alongside the participant so that if he/she loses balance, the instructor is there to help; hand must remain on the hips, participant may not give baby steps

Appendix D continues on the next page →

Test 8	Modified curl-up
Purpose	To assess abdominal strength and endurance.
Equipment	Gymnasium mat.
Procedure	The participant lies in a supine position with knees bent and feet flat on the floor, and hands on thighs. During the curl-up, the participant slides his or her hands up the thighs to the superior part of the kneecap and then returns to the starting position. The fingers have to slide at least 10 cm along the legs to the kneecaps. The instructor's hands should be placed on the superior aspect of the kneecap, thereby assisting the participant in performing the correct technique. Fingers are not allowed to lift off the legs and the hands have to slide up simultaneously to the left and right kneecap, respectively (one hand should not lead the other). The participant should perform as many curl-ups as possible (up to a maximum of 75). The rate or pace of the curl-up should be one curl-up every 3 s. The instructor should verbally count the number of curl-ups. Only one trial is administered. A practice trial of less than three curl-ups should be implemented. *Source*: Drawing published with permission from the artist, Luibov Mazanko, *c.* 2013-2015, Port Elizabeth, South Africa.
Scoring	Number of curl-ups from starting position to the superior aspect of the knee cap.
Safety precautions and general instructions	Stop the test if pain is experienced. Ensure that the hands remain on the thighs throughout the movement. Hands should move up simultaneously. Motivation is key.

Appendix D continues on the next page →

Test 9	Trunk lift
Purpose	To assess trunk strength (see Figure A-8).
Equipment	Ruler 50 cm in length and gymnasium mat.
Procedure	From a prone position with hands under the thighs, the participant should attempt to lift their chins up to a maximum height from the mat by arching the back. The measurement is taken with a tape measure from the mat to the bottom of the chin (lower jaw). Ensure that the ruler is vertically straight. Two trials are allowed and the best score is noted. *Source*: Drawing published with permission from the artist, Luibov Mazanko, *c.* 2013-2015, Port Elizabeth, South Africa.
Scoring	Distance from the mat to the bottom of the chin (lower jaw) in cm.
Safety precautions and general instructions	Stop the test if pain is experienced. Ensure that the hands remain under the thighs.

Appendix D continues on the next page →

Test 10	30-second chair stand test
Purpose	To assess lower body strength.
Equipment	Folding chair with a seat height of 43 cm (17 inches) and stopwatch.
Procedure	Participants sit on a straight-backed chair (43 cm in height and with no arm rests), feet flat on the floor and arms across the chest. On the signal 'go', the participant rises to a full stand and returns to a fully seated position. Before testing, the participant performs two or three stands to ensure the correct technique. Every time the person sits, the back (positioned upright and straight) should touch the back of the chair. Two trials are administered.

Source: Drawing published with permission from the artist, Luibov Mazanko, c. 2013-2015, Port Elizabeth, South Africa.

Scoring	The score is the number of stands completed in 30 s. If the person is more than halfway up at the end of the 30 s, it counts as a full stand.
Safety precautions and general instructions	Place the chair against the wall to prevent falling. Stand close to the chair in case the participant loses his or her balance. Stop the test if pain is experienced. Motivation is key.

Appendix D continues on the next page →

Test 11	Handgrip strength
Purpose	To assess forearm and handgrip strength.
Equipment	Handgrip dynamometer and folding chair with no arm rests.
Procedure	Handgrip strength is assessed by a grip dynamometer with a grip space of 10 cm. Participants sit on a straight-backed chair without arms, feet flat on the floor. The elbow is flexed at 90° and the grip dynamometer is squeezed as hard as possible. Three trials are administered, with 30 s rest in between each trial. Both hands are tested. The best score for each hand is recorded. *Source*: Drawing published with permission from the artist, Luibov Mazanko, *c.* 2013-2015, Port Elizabeth, South Africa.
Scoring	The device digitally recorded the participant's test score (kg).
Safety precautions and general instructions	-

Appendix D continues on the next page →

Test 12	Isometric push-up
Purpose	To assess upper body endurance.
Equipment	Stopwatch.
Procedure	Participants attempt to hold the push-up position for as long as they can. Hands are placed directly below the shoulders with arms extended. The back has to be perfectly aligned with the rest of the body and toes have to be on the floor. The time that the position is held is recorded to the nearest second. Only one trial is administered. A practice session for 3–5 s may be attempted to ensure proper posture. Time is stopped as soon as the back sags or lifts. Proper form is to be strictly controlled. *Source*: Drawing published with permission from the artist, Luibov Mazanko, c. 2013-2015, Port Elizabeth, South Africa.
Scoring	Amount of time (in seconds) that the proper form of the push-up position is maintained.
Safety precautions and general instructions	Stop the test if pain is experienced. Motivation is key. Proper form (no sagging or lifting of the back) is important.

Test 13	6-minute walk distance test
Purpose	To assess aerobic endurance whilst walking.
Equipment	Cones, measuring tape and stopwatch.
Procedure	The participant walks as fast as possible in a rectangle (perimeter 50 yards [20 yards by 5 yards]) for 6 min. For improved accuracy and pacing, participants should practice this test, the day before the test. On the signal 'go', the participant attempts to walk as many laps as possible within 6 min. No running is allowed. To assist with pacing, participants should be alerted every time a minute has elapsed. A 1:1 pacer was provided, as has been described in adults with ID by Nasuti, Stuart-Hill and Temple (2013).
	No image.

Appendix D continues on the next page →

Scoring	Convert the number of laps walked (rounded to the nearest quarter, halve, or three quarters or full lap) to the distance in yards or metres. Only one trial is administered.
Safety precautions and general instructions	Stop the test if pain, dizziness, chest pain, heart palpitations or any form of sign or symptom contraindicated to exercise is experienced. Motivation is key. No running is allowed.

Test 14	16-metre PACER test
Purpose	To assess aerobic endurance (running).
Equipment	Cones, measuring tape, CD player and PACER CD.
Procedure	At the sound of a tape-recorded beep, participants run from one line (cone) to the other, 16 m away. If the participant fails to reach the line before the beep, a warning is provided. If he/she fails to reach the line again, the test is stopped. Only one trial is given. The test instructor should run alongside the participant (1:1 PACER). The sound of the tape-recorded beep increases in pace as the test progresses. **16m** *Source*: Drawing published with permission from the artist, Luibov Mazanko, c. 2013-2015, Port Elizabeth, South Africa.
Scoring	The test score was the number of laps completed on pace.
Safety precautions and general instructions	Stop the test if pain, dizziness, chest pain, heart palpitations or any form of sign or symptom contraindicated to exercise is experienced. It is advised that a health professional is present during this test. Motivation is key. Ensure that the participant does not lose his or her balance during running or turning. Monitor participants for overexertion.

Appendix E: Participant raw scorecard

Personal information				
Name:		**Surname:**		
Gender:		**Age:**		
Level of education:		**Type of DS:**		
Living arrangement:	Care centre or private	**Physical activity:**	/week	
Body mass and height (two tests)				
Height:	cm	**Body mass:**		kg
Functional fitness (12 tests)				

Aerobic tests (two tests)					
6-minute walk distance		laps		metres	
16-metre PACER		level		shuttles	

Flexibility (2 tests)							
Chair sit-and-reach test	Left leg:	Trial 1:	cm	Trial 2:		cm	
	Right leg:	Trial 1:	cm	Trial 2:		cm	
Back scratch test	Left shoulder:	Trial 1:	cm	Trial 2:		cm	
	Right shoulder:	Trial 1:	cm	Trial 2:		cm	

Muscular strength and endurance (five tests)									
Handgrip strength	Left hand	Trial 1:	kg	Trial 2:	kg	Trial 3:	kg		
	Right hand	Trial 1:	kg	Trial 2:	kg	Trial 3:	kg		
Isometric push-up		Trial 1:	sec						
Trunk lift		Trial 1:	cm	Trial 2:		cm			
Modified curl-up		Trial 1:	amount						
30-second chair stand test		Trial 1:	amount	Trial 2:		amount			

Balance (two tests)						
Standing on one leg	Left leg	Trial 1:	sec	Trial 2:		sec
	Right leg	Trial 1:	sec	Trial 2:		sec
Walking on the balance beam		Trial 1:	steps	Trial 2:		steps

Functional Test					
8-foot up-and-go test	Trial 1:	sec	Trial 2:		sec

Appendix F: Final scorecard and percentile norms

Personal information			
Name		Surname	
Gender		Age	
Physical activity (sessions per week)		Date of test	

Body mass and height					
Height (cm)		Body mass (kg)		BMI (kg/m²)	

Functional fitness tests				
Test		Test score	Percentile	Meet minimum requirements
1. Flexibility	1.1. Chair sit-and-reach test (n) (RS)			
	1.2. Back scratch test (cm) (RS)			
2. Functional ability	2.1. 8-foot up-and-go (s)			
3. Balance	3.1. Standing on one leg (s) (RS)			
	3.2. Walking on balance beam (steps)			
4. Muscular strength and endurance	4.1. Modified curl-up (n)			
	4.2. Trunk lift (cm)			
	4.3. 30-second chair stand test (n)			
	4.4. Handgrip strength (kg) (RS)			
	4.5. Isometric push-up (s)			
5. Aerobic tests	5.1. 6-minute walk distance test (m)			
	5.2. 16-metre PACER (shuttles)			

RS, right-hand side.

Appendix G: Adapted physical activity readiness questionnaire

Regular physical activity is fun and healthy and more people should increase their physical activity every day. Being more physically active is very safe for MOST people.
Please read the questions carefully and answer each one honestly. If you have any concerns about your health status, you should check with your doctor before becoming more physically active.

Question		Yes	No
1	Has your doctor ever said that you have a heart condition OR high blood pressure?		
2	Do you feel pain in your chest at rest, during your daily activities of living, OR when you do physical activity?		
3	Do you lose balance because of dizziness OR have you lost consciousness (fainted) in the last 12 months?		
4	Have you ever been diagnosed by a health professional as having any of the following (Check all that apply)?		

Heart trouble	Arthritis	Back problems
High blood pressure	Chronic asthma	Foot problems
High cholesterol	Emphysema	Allergies
Diabetes	Bronchitis	Trouble hearing

Question			Yes	No
5	Are you currently taking any medication for any of the conditions listed above?	*Please describe:*		
6	Do you have a bone or joint problem that could be made worse by becoming more physically active? (if you had a joint problem in the past, e.g. knee, ankle and shoulder, please answer NO to this question).			

Appendix G continues on the next page →

7	Has your Doctor, Nurse Practitioner (or health provider) ever said that you should only do medically supervised physical activity?		

Acknowledgement		
8	I have read and understood the above health questions and directions regarding my participation in the Fit, Fun & Fully Alive! Group Fitness Classes.	Your Initials _____

Disclaimer
IF YOU ANSWERED YES to one or more of the questions above, you should consult your doctor or health provider first before becoming more physically active. Talk with your doctor about the kinds of activities you wish to participate in and follow his or her advice.
IF YOU ANSWERED NO to all the questions above, you can be reasonably sure that you can start becoming more physically active.   • Begin slowly and build up gradually. Delay becoming more active if you are not feeling well because of a temporary illness such as a cold or a fever wait until you feel better.   • If your health changes so that you would answer YES to any of the PAR-Q questions, ask for advice from your health professional and let your Fitness Instructor know.

Appendix H: How to use the functional fitness battery test

FUNCTIONAL FITNESS BATTERY TEST	
It is suggested that the participant follows the following steps:	
1	The participant visits his primary health care practitioner with the adapted physical activity readiness questionnaire (attached as an appendix) to verify whether he or she is ready to perform physical activity test (app. G).
2	An academic researcher or exercise specialist with experience in working with adults with DS should carefully study the contents presented in this book. Especially, the methodology section should be carefully studied (ch. 4).
3	The academic researcher or adapted physical activity specialist should obtain the page outlining equipment needed (Appendix C), order of tests and stations (Appendix D), and the participant score sheet (app. E).
4	The academic researcher or adapted physical activity exercise specialist sets up the test venue with equipment as stipulated in Appendixes D and E.
5	The adapted physical activity specialist provides the participant and his or her parent or guardian with the consent form, as well as a short verbal and physical description and demonstration of all the tests involved in this book. The activity specialist also provides the participant with the form of important information pertaining to 24 h before the test (Appendix B). After a minimum of 5 days that have elapsed, the informed consent form is collected. The activity specialist and the participant's parent or guardian identify an appropriate day for exercise testing to commence at 09:00 in the morning.
6	On testing day, the adapted physical activity specialist proceeds to perform a basic warm-up with the participant where the major muscle groups are exercised and stretched. Content in Chapter 5 provides some examples and guidelines.
7	The academic researcher or adapted physical activity exercise specialist instructs participant to complete all 14 tests. The contents of Chapter 4 and the information provided in Appendix D provide clear guidelines. The 6-minute distance walk test is always performed at last. The 16-metre shuttle run test is always performed on the following day
8	The participant's test score is recorded and compared with the normative tables found in Chapter 3. Whether the participants' test score reaches minimal acceptable standards should also be recorded. See bolded rows in the various tables.
9	The adapted physical activity exercise specialist provides the participant with exercises to maintain existing strengths and improve weaknesses (ch. 6).
10	The participant should be re-assessed after a period of 3 months to monitor progress of the exercise intervention.

References

Abbag, F.I., 2006, 'Congenital heart diseases and other major anomalies in patients with Down syndrome', *Saudi Medical Journal* 27(2), 219–222.

Abizanda, P., Navarro, J.L., García-Tomás, M.I., López-Jiménez, E., Martínez-Sánchez, E. & Paterna, G., 2012, 'Validity and usefulness of hand-held dynamometry for measuring muscle strength in community-dwelling older persons', *Archives of Gerontology and Geriatrics* 54(1), 21–27. https://doi.org/10.1016/j.archger.2011.02.006

American Alliance for Health, Physical Education, and Recreation, 1976, *Special fitness test manual for mildly mentally retarded persons*, American Alliance for Health, Physical Education, and Recreation, Washington, DC.

American Alliance for Health, Physical Education, Recreation and Dance, 1978, *Special fitness test manual*, American Alliance for Health, Physical Education, Recreation and Dance, Washington, DC.

American College of Sports Medicine (ACSM), 2013, *ACSM's guidelines for exercise testing and prescription*, 9th edn., Lippincott Williams & Wilkins, Baltimore, MD.

Arena, R., Myers, J., Williams, M.A., Gulati, M., Kligfield, P., Balady, G.J. et al., 2007, 'Assessment of functional capacity in clinical and research settings: A scientific statement from the American Heart Association committee on exercise, rehabilitation, and prevention of the council on clinical cardiology and the council on cardiovascular nursing', *Circulation* 116(3), 329–343. https://doi.org/10.1161/CIRCULATIONAHA.106.184461

Baptista, F., Varela, A. & Sardinha, L.B., 2005, 'Bone mineral mass in males and females with and without Down syndrome', *Osteoporosis International* 16(4), 380–388. https://doi.org/10.1007/s00198-004-1687-1

Barnhart, R.C. & Connolly, B., 2007, 'Aging and Down syndrome: Implications for physical therapy', *Physical Therapy* 87(10), 1399–1406. https://doi.org/10.2522/ptj.20060334

Barr, M. & Shields, N., 2011, 'Identifying the barriers and facilitators to participation in physical activity for children with Down syndrome', *Journal of Intellectual Disability Research* 55(11), 1020–1033. https://doi.org/10.1111/j.1365-2788.2011.01425.x

Bassey, E.J., Morgan, K., Dallosso, H.M. & Ebrahim, S.B.J., 1989, 'Flexibility of the shoulder joint measured as range of abduction in a large representative sample of men and women over 65 years of age', *European Journal of Applied Physiology and Occupational Physiology* 58(4), 353–360. https://doi.org/10.1007/BF00643509

Baynard, T., Pitetti, K.H., Guerra, M. & Fernhall, B., 2004, 'Heart rate variability at rest and during exercise in persons with Down syndrome', *Archives of Physical Medicine and Rehabilitation* 85(8), 1285–1290. https://doi.org/10.1016/j.apmr.2003.11.023

Baynard, T., Pitetti, K.H., Guerra, M., Unnithan, V.B. & Fernhall, B., 2008, 'Age-related changes in aerobic capacity in individuals with mental retardation: A 20-yr review', *Medicine and Science in Sports and Exercise* 40(11), 1984–1989. https://doi.org/10.1249/MSS.0b013e31817f19a1

Bertapelli, F., Pitetti, K., Agiovlasitis, S. & Guerra-Junior, G., 2016, 'Overweight and obesity in children and adolescents with Down syndrome – Prevalence, determinants, consequences, and interventions: A literature review', *Research in Developmental Disabilities* 57, 181–192. https://doi.org/10.1016/j.ridd.2016.06.018

Bittles, A.H. & Glasson, E.J., 2004, 'Clinical, social, and ethical implications of changing life expectancy in Down syndrome', *Developmental Medicine and Child Neurology* 46(4), 282–286. https://doi.org/10.1111/j.1469-8749.2004.tb00483.x

Bittles, A.H., Petterson, B.A., Sullivan, S.G., Hussain, R., Glasson, E.J. & Montgomery, P.D., 2002, 'The influence of intellectual disability on life expectancy', *The Journals of Gerontology*

Series A: Biological Sciences and Medical Sciences 57(7), 470–472. https://doi.org/10.1093/gerona/57.7.M470

Bocalini, D.S., Santos, L.D. & Serra, A.J., 2008, 'Physical exercise improves the functional capacity and quality of life in patients with heart failure', *Clinics* 63(4), 437–442. https://doi.org/10.1590/S1807-59322008000400005

Boer, P.H., 2010, 'The functional fitness capacity of adults with Down syndrome in South Africa', Masters thesis, Department of Sport Science, Stellenbosch University.

Boer, P.H., 2015, 'Effect of continuous aerobic vs interval training on selected functional fitness parameters of adults with intellectual disability and Down syndrome', PhD thesis, Physical Activity, Sport and Recreation, North-West University.

Boer, P.H., 2017, 'Effects of detraining on anthropometry, aerobic capacity and functional ability in adults with Down syndrome', *Special Issue: Physical Health* 31(5), 144–150. https://doi.org/10.1111/jar.12327

Boer, P.H., 2020, 'The effect of 8 weeks of freestyle swim training on the functional fitness of adults with Down syndrome', *Journal of Intellectual Disability Research* 64(10), 770–781. https://doi.org/10.1111/jir.12768

Boer, P.H. & De Beer, Z., 2019, 'The effect of aquatic exercises on the physical and functional fitness of adults with Down syndrome: A non-randomised controlled trial', *Journal of Intellectual Disability Research* 63(12), 1453–1463. https://doi.org/10.1111/jir.12687

Boer, P.H., Meeus, M., Terblanche, E., Rombaut, L., Wandele, I.D., Hermans, L. et al., 2014, 'The influence of sprint interval training on body composition, physical and metabolic fitness in adolescents and young adults with intellectual disability: A randomized controlled trial', *Clinical Rehabilitation* 28(3), 221–231. https://doi.org/10.1177/0269215513498609

Boer, P.H. & Moss, S.J., 2016a, 'Effect of continuous aerobic vs. interval training on selected anthropometrical, physiological and functional parameters of adults with Down syndrome', *Journal of Intellectual Disability Research* 60(4), 322–334. https://doi.org/10.1111/jir.12251

Boer, P.H. & Moss, S.J., 2016b, 'Test–retest reliability and minimal detectable change scores of twelve functional fitness tests in adults with Down syndrome', *Research in Developmental Disabilities* 48, 176–185. https://doi.org/10.1016/j.ridd.2015.10.022

Boer, P.H. & Moss, S.J., 2016c, 'Validity of the 16-metre PACER and six-minute walk test in adults with Down syndrome', *Disability and Rehabilitation* 38(26), 2575–2583. https://doi.org/10.3109/09638288.2015.1137982

Bohannon, R.W., 1998, 'Alternatives for measuring knee extension strength of the elderly at home', *Clinical Rehabilitation* 12(5), 434–440. https://doi.org/10.1191/026921598673062266

Brill, P., 2004, *Functional fitness for older adults*, Human Kinetics, Champaign, IL.

Cabeza-Ruiz, R., García-Massó, X., Centeno-Prada, R.A., Beas-Jiménez, J.D., Colado, J.C. & González, L.M., 2011, 'Time and frequency analysis of the static balance in young adults with Down syndrome', *Gait & Posture* 33(1), 23–28. https://doi.org/10.1016/j.gaitpost.2010.09.014

Carfi, A., Antocicco, M., Brandi, V., Cipriani, C., Fiore, F., Mascia, D. et al., 2014, 'Characteristics of adults with Down syndrome: Prevalence of age-related conditions', *Frontiers in Medicine* 1, 51–59. https://doi.org/10.3389/fmed.2014.00051

Carmeli, E., Kessel, S., Bar-Chad, S. & Merrick, J., 2004, 'A comparison between older persons with Down syndrome and a control group: Clinical characteristics, functional status and sensori-motor function', *Downs Syndrome Research and Practice* 9(1), 17–24.

Carmeli, E., Kessel, S., Coleman, R. & Ayalon, M., 2002, 'Effects of a treadmill walking program on muscle strength and balance in elderly people with Down syndrome', *The Journals of Gerontology Series A: Biological Sciences and Medical Sciences* 57(2), 106–110. https://doi.org/10.1093/gerona/57.2.M106

Carmeli, E., Zinger-Vaknin, T., Morad, M. & Merrick, J., 2005, 'Can physical training have an effect on well-being in adults with mild intellectual disability?', *Mechanisms of Ageing and Development* 126(2), 299–304. https://doi.org/10.1016/j.mad.2004.08.021

Casey, A.F., Wang, X. & Osterling, K., 2012, 'Test-retest reliability of the 6-minute walk test in individuals with Down syndrome', *Archives of Physical Medicine and Rehabilitation* 93(11), 2068–2074. https://doi.org/10.1016/j.apmr.2012.04.022

Chakravarty, K. & Webley, M., 1993, 'Shoulder joint movement and its relationship to disability in the elderly', *The Journal of Rheumatology* 20(8), 1359–1361.

Chalise, H.N., Saito, T. & Kai, I., 2008, 'Functional disability in activities of daily living and instrumental activities of daily living among Nepalese Newar elderly', *Public Health* 122(4), 394–396. https://doi.org/10.1016/j.puhe.2007.07.015

Chen, C.C.J., Ringenbach, D.R.S. & Snow, M., 2014, 'Treadmill walking effects on grip strength in young men with Down syndrome', *Research in Developmental Disabilities* 35(2), 288–293. https://doi.org/10.1016/j.ridd.2013.10.032

Chiang, D.J., Pritchard, M.T. & Nagy, L.E., 2011, 'Obesity, diabetes mellitus, and liver fibrosis', *American Journal of Physiology* 300(5), G697–G702. https://doi.org/10.1152/ajpgi.00426.2010

Chicoine, B. & McGuire, D., 1997, 'Longevity of a woman with Down syndrome: A case study', *Mental Retardation* 35(6), 477–479. https://doi.org/10.1352/0047-6765(1997)035%3C0477:LOAWWD%3E2.0.CO;2

Cowley, P.M., Ploutz-Snyder, L.L., Baynard, T., Heffernan, K., Jae, S.Y. & Hsu, S., 2010, 'Physical fitness predicts functional tasks in individuals with Down syndrome', *Medicine & Science in Sports & Exercise* 42(2), 388–393. https://doi.org/10.1249/MSS.0b013e3181b07e7a

Cowley, P.M., Ploutz-Snyder, L.L., Baynard, T., Heffernan, K.S., Jae, S.Y., Hsu, S. et al., 2011, 'The effect of progressive resistance training on leg strength, aerobic capacity and functional tasks of daily living in persons with Down syndrome', *Disability & Rehabilitation* 33(22), 2229–2236. https://doi.org/10.3109/09638288.2011.563820

De Asua, D.R., Quero, M., Moldenhauer, F. & Suarez, C., 2015, 'Clinical profile and main comorbidities of Spanish adults with Down syndrome', *European Journal of Internal Medicine* 26(6), 385–391. https://doi.org/10.1016/j.ejim.2015.05.003

Dodd, K.J. & Shields, N., 2005, 'A systematic review of the outcomes of cardiovascular exercise programs for people with Down syndrome', *Archives of Physical Medicine and Rehabilitation* 86(10), 2051–2058. https://doi.org/10.1016/j.apmr.2005.06.003

Down Syndrome South Africa, 2020, 'Working to improve the lives of people with Down syndrome', viewed 25 April 2020, from http://www.downsyndrome.org.za.

Eberhard, Y., Eterradossi, J. & Rapacchi, B., 1989, 'Physical aptitudes to exertion in children with Down's syndrome', *Journal of Intellectual Disability Research* 33(2), 167–174. https://doi.org/10.1111/j.1365-2788.1989.tb01463.x

Elmahgoub, S.S., Van de Velde, A., Peersman, W., Cambier, D. & Calders, P., 2012, 'Reproducibility, validity and predictors of six-minute walk test in overweight and obese adolescents with intellectual disability', *Disability and Rehabilitation* 34(10), 846–851. https://doi.org/10.3109/09638288.2011.623757

Esposito, P.E., MacDonald, M., Hornyak, J.E. & Ulrich, D.A., 2012, 'Physical activity patterns of youth with Down syndrome', *Intellectual and Developmental Disabilities* 50(2), 109–119. https://doi.org/10.1352/1934-9556-50.2.109

Fait, H.F. & Dunn, J.M., 1984, *FAIT physical fitness test for mildly and moderately mentally retarded students*, Saunders College, Philadelphia, PA.

Fernhall, B., Millar, A.L., Tymeson, G.T. & Burkett, L.N., 1990, 'Maximal exercise testing of mentally retarded adolescents and adults: Reliability study', *Archives of Physical Medicine and Rehabilitation* 71(13), 1065–1068.

Fernhall, B. & Pitetti, K.H., 2001, 'Limitations to physical work capacity in individuals with mental retardation', *Clinical Exercise Physiology* 3(4), 176–185.

Fernhall, B., Pitetti, K.H., Rimmer, J.H., McCubbin, J.A., Rintala, P., Millar, A.L., Kittredge, J. & Burkett, L.N., 1996, 'Cardiorespiratory capacity of individuals with mental retardation including

Down syndrome', *Medicine and Science in Sports and Exercise* 28(3), 366–371. https://doi.org/10.1249/00005768-199603000-00012

Fernhall, B., Pitetti, K.H., Vukovich, M.D., Stubbs, N., Hensen, T., Winnick, J.P. et al., 1998, 'Validation of cardiovascular fitness field tests in children with mental retardation', *American Journal Mental Retardation* 102(6), 602–612. https://doi.org/10.1352/0895-8017(1998)102%3C0602:VOCFFT%3E2.0.CO;2

Folin, M., Baiguera, S., Conconi, M.T., Pati, T., Grandi, C., Parnigotto, P.P. & Nussdorfer, G.G., 2003, 'The impact of risk factors of Alzheimer's disease in the Down syndrome', *International Journal of Molecular Medicine* 11(2), 267–270. https://doi.org/10.3892/ijmm.11.2.267

Galli, M., Rigoldi, C., Mainardi, L., Tenore, N., Onorati, P. & Albertini, G., 2008, 'Postural control in patients with Down syndrome', *Disability and Rehabilitation* 30(17), 1274–1278. https://doi.org/10.1080/09638280701610353

González-Agüero, A., Vicente-Rodríguez, G., Gómez-Cabello, A., Ara, I., Moreno, L.A. & Casajús, J.A., 2011, 'A combined training intervention programme increases lean mass in youths with Down syndrome', *Research in Developmental Disabilities* 32(6), 2383–2388. https://doi.org/10.1016/j.ridd.2011.07.024

González-Agüero, A., Vicente-Rodríguez, G., Moreno, L.A., Guerra-Balic, M., Ara, I. & Casajús, J.A., 2010, 'Health-related physical fitness in children and adolescents with Down syndrome and response to training', *Scandinavian Journal of Medicine & Science in Sports* 20(5), 716–724. https://doi.org/10.1111/j.1600-0838.2010.01120.x

Goodman, C.C. & Miedaner, J., 1998, *Genetic and developmental disorders*, WB Saunders, Philadelphia, PA.

Guerra, M., Pitetti, K.H. & Fernhall, B., 2003, 'Cross validation of the 20-meter shuttle run test for adolescents with Down syndrome', *Adapted Physical Activity Quarterly* 20(1), 70–79. https://doi.org/10.1123/apaq.20.1.70

Guerra-Balic, M., Oviedo, G.R., Javierre, C., Fortuno, J., Barnet-Lopez, S., Nino, O. et al., 2015, 'Reliability and validity of the 6-min walk test in adults and seniors with intellectual disabilities', *Research in Developmental Disabilities* 47, 144–153. https://doi.org/10.1016/j.ridd.2015.09.011

Gupta, S., Rao, B.K. & Sd, K., 2011, 'Effect of strength and balance training in children with Down's syndrome: A randomized controlled trial', *Clinical Rehabilitation* 25(5), 425–432. https://doi.org/10.1177/0269215510382929

Heller, T., Hsieh, K. & Rimmer, J., 2003, 'Barriers and supports for exercise participation among adults with Down syndrome', *Journal of Gerontology Social Work* 38(2), 161–178. https://doi.org/10.1300/J083v38n01_03

Heller, T., Hsieh, K. & Rimmer, J.H., 2004, 'Attitudinal and psychosocial outcomes of a fitness and health education program on adults with Down syndrome', *American Journal on Mental Retardation* 109(2), 175–185. https://doi.org/10.1352/0895-8017(2004)109%3C175:AAPOOA%3E2.0.CO;2

Hermon, C., Alberman, E., Beral, V. & Swerdlow, A., 2001, 'Mortality and cancer incidence in persons with Down's syndrome, their parents and siblings', *Annals of Human Genetics* 65(2), 167–176. https://doi.org/10.1046/j.1469-1809.2001.6520167.x

Hilgenkamp, T.I., Van Wijck, R. & Evenhuis, H.M., 2010, 'Physical fitness in older people with ID – Concept and measuring instruments: A review', *Research in Developmental Disabilities* 31(5), 1027–1038. https://doi.org/10.1016/j.ridd.2010.04.012

Hilgenkamp, T.I., Van Wijck, R. & Evenhuis, H.M., 2012, 'Feasibility and reliability of physical fitness tests in older adults with intellectual disability: A pilot study', *Journal of Intellectual and Developmental Disability* 37(2), 158–162. https://doi.org/10.3109/13668250.2012.681773

Hilgenkamp, T.I., Van Wijck, R. & Evenhuis, H.M., 2013, 'Feasibility of eight physical fitness tests in 1,050 older adults with intellectual disability: Results of the healthy ageing with intellectual disabilities study', *Intellectual and Developmental Disabilities* 51(1), 33–47. https://doi.org/10.1352/1934-9556-51.01.033

Iacobellis, G., Ribaudo, M.C., Zappaterreno, A., Lannucci, C.V. & Leonetti, F., 2005, 'Prevalence of uncomplicated obesity in an Italian obese population', *Obesity Research* 13(6), 1116–1122. https://doi.org/10.1038/oby.2005.130

Irving, C., Basu, A., Richmond, S., Burn, J. & Wren, C., 2008, 'Twenty-year trends in prevalence and survival of Down syndrome', *European Journal of Human Genetics* 16(11), 1336–1340. https://doi.org/10.1038/ejhg.2008.122

Izzo, A., Mollo, N., Nitti, M., Paladino, S., Calì, G., Genesio, R. et al., 2018, 'Mitochondrial dysfunction in Down syndrome: Molecular mechanisms and therapeutic targets', *Molecular Medicine* 24(1), 1–8. https://doi.org/10.1186/s10020-018-0004-y

Johnson, L. & Londeree, B., 1976, *Motor fitness testing manual for the moderately mentally retarded*, American Alliance for Health, Physical Education and Recreation, Washington, DC.

Jones, C.J., Rikli, R.E. & Beam, W.C., 1999, 'A 30-s chair-stand test as a measure of lower body strength in community-residing older adults', *Research Quarterly for Exercise and Sport* 70(2), 113–119. https://doi.org/10.1080/02701367.1999.10608028

Jones, C.J., Rikli, R.E., Max, J. & Noffal, G., 1998, 'The reliability and validity of a chair sit-and-reach test as a measure of hamstring flexibility in older adults', *Research Quarterly Exercise and Sport* 69(4), 338–343. https://doi.org/10.1080/02701367.1998.10607708

Kenney, W., Wilmore, J. & Costill, D., 2015, *Physiology of sport and exercise*, Human Kinetics, Champaign, IL.

Kerstiens, R.L. & Green, M., 2015, 'Exercise in individuals with Down syndrome: A brief review', *International Journal of Exercise Science* 8(2), 192–201.

Krinsky-McHale, S.J., Devenny, D.A. & Silverman, W.P., 2002, 'Changes in explicit memory associated with early dementia in adults with Down's syndrome', *Journal of Intellectual Disability Research* 46(3), 198–208. https://doi.org/10.1046/j.1365-2788.2002.00365.x

Lewis, C.L. & Fragala-Pinkham, M.A., 2005, 'Effects of aerobic conditioning and strength training on a child with Down syndrome: A case study', *Pediatric Physical Therapy* 17(1), 30–36. https://doi.org/10.1097/01.PEP.0000154185.55735.A0

Lin, M.R., Hwang, H.F., Hu, M.H., Wu, H.D.I., Wang, Y.W. & Huang, F.C., 2004, 'Psychometric comparisons of the timed up and go, one-leg stand, functional reach, and Tinetti balance measures in community-dwelling older people', *Journal of the American Geriatrics Society* 52(8), 1343–1348. https://doi.org/10.1111/j.1532-5415.2004.52366.x

Lobelo, F., Stoutenberg, M. & Hutber, A., 2014, 'The exercise is medicine global health initiative: A 2014 update', *British Journal of Sports Medicine* 48(22), 1627–1633. https://doi.org/10.1136/bjsports-2013-093080

Loovis, E.M. & Ersing, W.F., 1979, *Assessing and programming gross motor development for children*, Ohio Motor Assessment Associates, Cleveland Heights, OH.

Mahy, J., Shields, N., Taylor, N.F. & Dodd, K.J., 2010, 'Identifying facilitators and barriers to physical activity for adults with Down syndrome', *Journal of Intellectual Disability Research* 54(9), 795–805. https://doi.org/10.1111/j.1365-2788.2010.01308.x

Melville, C., Cooper, S., Morrison, J., Allan, L., Smiley, E. & Williamson, A., 2008, 'The prevalence and determinants of obesity in adults with intellectual disabilities', *Journal of Applied Research in Intellectual Disabilities* 21(5), 425–437. https://doi.org/10.1111/j.1468-3148.2007.00412.x

Mendonca, G.V. & Pereira, F.D., 2009, 'Influence of long-term exercise training on submaximal and peak aerobic capacity and locomotor economy in adult males with Down's syndrome', *Medical Science Monitor: International Medical Journal of Experimental and Clinical Research* 15(2), 33–39.

Mendonca, G.V., Pereira, F.D. & Fernhall, B., 2011, 'Effects of combined aerobic and resistance exercise training in adults with and without Down syndrome', *Archives of Physical Medicine and Rehabilitation* 92(1), 37–45. https://doi.org/10.1016/j.apmr.2010.09.015

Mendonca, G.V., Pereira, F.D. & Fernhall, B., 2013, 'Heart rate recovery and variability following combined aerobic and resistance exercise training in adults with and without Down syndrome', *Research in Developmental Disabilities* 34(1), 353–361. https://doi.org/10.1016/j.ridd.2012.08.023

Meredith, M. & Welk, G., 2010, *Fitnessgram and activitygram test administration manual-updated*, 4th edn., Human Kinetics, Champaign, IL.

Millán-Calenti, J.C., Tubío, J., Pita-Fernández, S., González-Abraldes, I., Lorenzo, T., Fernández-Arruty, T. et al., 2010, 'Prevalence of functional disability in activities of daily living (ADL), instrumental activities of daily living (IADL) and associated factors, as predictors of morbidity and mortality', *Archives of Gerontology and Geriatrics* 50(3), 306–310. https://doi.org/10.1016/j.archger.2009.04.017

Moore, G., Durstine, J.L., Painter, P. & American College of Sports Medicine, 2016, *ACSM's exercise management for persons with chronic diseases & disabilities*, Human Kinetics, Champaign, IL.

Morey, M.C., Pieper, C.F. & Cornoni-Huntley, J., 1998, 'Physical fitness and functional limitations in community-dwelling older adults', *Medicine & Science in Sports & Exercise* 30(5), 715–723. https://doi.org/10.1097/00005768-199805000-00012

Mutton, D. & Alberman, E., 1996, 'Cytogenetic and epidemiological findings in Down syndrome, England and Wales 1989 to 1993. National Down Syndrome Cytogenetic Register and the Association', *Journal of Medical Genetics* 33(5), 387–394. https://doi.org/10.1136/jmg.33.5.387

Nasuti, G., Stuart-Hill, L. & Temple, V.A., 2013, 'The six-minute walk test for adults with intellectual disability: A study of validity and reliability', *Journal of Intellectual and Developmental Disability* 38(1), 31–38. https://doi.org/10.3109/13668250.2012.748885

National Down Syndrome Society, 2020, *The national advocate for the value, acceptance, inclusion of people with Down syndrome*, viewed 25 April 2020, from http://www.ndss.org.

Niemann, B., Chen, Y., Teschner, M., Li, L., Silber, R.E. & Rohrbach, S., 2011, 'Obesity induces signs of premature cardiac aging in younger patients: The role of mitochondria', *Journal of the American College of Cardiology* 57(5), 577–585. https://doi.org/10.1016/j.jacc.2010.09.040

Nordstrøm, M., Hansen, B.H., Paus, B. & Kolset, S.O., 2013, 'Accelerometer-determined physical activity and walking capacity in persons with Down syndrome, Williams syndrome and Prader-Willi syndrome', *Research in Developmental Disabilities* 34(12), 4395–4403. https://doi.org/10.1016/j.ridd.2013.09.021

Oeser, A., Chung, C.P., Asanuma, Y., Avalos, I. & Stein, C.M., 2005, 'Obesity is an independent contributor to functional capacity and inflammation in systemic lupus erythematosus', *Arthritis & Rheumatism* 52(11), 3651–3659. https://doi.org/10.1002/art.21400

Oliver, C., Crayton, L., Holland, A., Hall, S. & Bradbury, J., 1998, 'A four year prospective study of age-related cognitive change in adults with Down's syndrome', *Psychological Medicine* 28(6), 1365–1377. https://doi.org/10.1017/S0033291798007417

Ordonez, F.J., Rosety, M. & Rosety-Rodriguez, M., 2006, 'Influence of 12-week exercise training on fat mass percentage in adolescents with Down syndrome', *Medical Science Monitor* 12(10), CR416–CR419.

Oviedo, G.R., Guerra-Balic, M., Baynard, T. & Javierre, C., 2014, 'Effects of aerobic, resistance and balance training in adults with intellectual disabilities', *Research in Developmental Disabilities* 35(11), 2624–2634. https://doi.org/10.1016/j.ridd.2014.06.025

Pataky, Z., Armand, S., Müller-Pinget, S., Golay, A. & Allet, L., 2014, 'Effects of obesity on functional capacity', *Obesity* 22(1), 56–62. https://doi.org/10.1002/oby.20514

Pescatello, L.S. & Riebe, D., 2014, *ACSM's guidelines for exercise testing and prescription*, Lippincott, Williams & Wilkins, Baltimore, MD.

Pikora, T.J., Bourke, J., Bathgate, K., Foley, K.R., Lennox, N. & Leonard, H., 2014, 'Health conditions and their impact among adolescents and young adults with Down syndrome', *PLoS One* 9(5), e96868. https://doi.org/10.1371/journal.pone.0096868

Pitetti, K.H., Baynard, T. & Agiovlasitis, S., 2013, 'Children and adolescents with Down syndrome, physical fitness and physical activity', *Journal of Sport and Health Science* 2(1), 47–57. https://doi.org/10.1016/j.jshs.2012.10.004

Pitetti, K.H. & Boneh, S., 1995, 'Cardiovascular fitness as related to leg strength in adults with mental retardation', *Medicine and Science in Sports and Exercise* 27(3), 423–428. https://doi.org/10.1249/00005768-199503000-00020

Pitetti, K.H. & Fernhall, B., 2004, 'Comparing run performance of adolescents with mental retardation, with and without Down syndrome', *Adapted Physical Activity Quarterly* 21(3), 219–228.

Podsiadlo, D. & Richardson, S., 1991, 'The timed "Up & Go": A test of basic functional mobility for frail elderly persons', *Journal of the American Geriatrics Society* 39(2), 142–148. https://doi.org/10.1111/j.1532-5415.1991.tb01616.x

Prasher, V.P. & Filer, A., 1995, 'Behavioural disturbance in people with Down's syndrome and dementia', *Journal of Intellectual Disability Research* 39(5), 432–436. https://doi.org/10.1111/j.1365-2788.1995.tb00547.x

Presson, A.P., Partyka, G., Jensen, K.M., Devine, O.J., Rasmussen, S.A., McCabe, L.L. et al., 2013, 'Current estimate of Down syndrome population prevalence in the United States', *Journal of Pediatrics* 163(4), 1163–1168. https://doi.org/10.1016/j.jpeds.2013.06.013

Reiman, M. & Manske, R., 2009, *Functional testing in human performance*, Human Kinetics, Champaign, IL.

Reinders, N., Bryden, P.J. & Fletcher, P.C., 2015, 'Dancing with Down syndrome: A phenomenological case study', *Research in Dance Education* 16(3), 291–307. https://doi.org/10.1080/14647893.2015.1036018

Rigoldi, C., Galli, M., Mainardi, L., Crivellini, M. & Albertini, G., 2011, 'Postural control in children, teenagers and adults with Down syndrome', *Research in Developmental Disabilities* 32(1), 170–175. https://doi.org/10.1016/j.ridd.2010.09.007

Rikli, R.E., 2000, 'Reliability, validity, and methodological issues in assessing physical activity in older adults', *Research Quarterly for Exercise and Sport* 71(2), 89–96. https://doi.org/10.1080/02701367.2000.11082791

Rikli, R.E. & Jones, C.J., 1998, 'The reliability and validity of a 6-minute walk test as a measure of physical endurance in older adults', *Journal of Aging and Physical Activity* 6(4), 363–375. https://doi.org/10.1123/japa.6.4.363

Rikli, R.E. & Jones, C.J., 1999, 'Functional fitness normative scores for community-residing older adults, ages 60–94', *Journal of Aging and Physical Activity* 7, 162–181. https://doi.org/10.1123/japa.7.2.162

Rikli, R.E. & Jones, C.J., 2013, *Senior fitness test manual*, Human Kinetics, Champaign, IL.

Rimmer, J.H., Braddock, D.A. & Pitetti, K.H., 1996, 'Research on physical activity and disability: An emerging national priority', *Medicine & Science in Sports & Exercise* 28(11), 1366–1372. https://doi.org/10.1097/00005768-199611000-00004

Rimmer, J.H., Heller, T., Wang, E. & Valerio, I., 2004, 'Improvements in physical fitness in adults with Down syndrome', *American Journal of Mental Retardation* 109(2), 165–174. https://doi.org/10.1352/0895-8017(2004)109%3C165:IIPFIA%3E2.0.CO;2

Rubin, S.S., Rimmer, J.H., Chicoine, B., Braddock, D. & McGuire, D.E., 1998, 'Overweight prevalence in persons with Down syndrome', *Mental Retardation* 36(3), 175–181. https://doi.org/10.1352/0047-6765(1998)036%3C0175:OPIPWD%3E2.0.CO;2

Salaun, L. & Berthouze-Aranda, S.E., 2012, 'Physical fitness and fatness in adolescents with intellectual disabilities', *Journal of Applied Research in Intellectual Disability* 25(3), 231–239. https://doi.org/10.1111/j.1468-3148.2012.00659.x

Saunders, M.V., 2017, 'Effect of participation in shallow-water movement through the use of a stationary pole on pain and well-being of older adult women with knee and or hip osteoarthritis', Doctoral dissertation, Indiana University, viewed 09 March 2021, from http://hdl.handle.net/2022/22677.

Shamas-Ud-Din, S., 2002, 'Genetics of Down's syndrome and Alzheimer's disease', *The British Journal of Psychiatry* 181(2), 167–172. https://doi.org/10.1192/bjp.181.2.167

Shields, N., Bruder, A., Taylor, N. & Angelo, T., 2011, 'Influencing physiotherapy student attitudes toward exercise for adolescents with Down syndrome', *Disability & Rehabilitation* 33(4), 360–366. https://doi.org/10.3109/09638288.2010.498550

Shields, N., Dodd, K.J. & Abblitt, C., 2009, 'Do children with Down syndrome perform sufficient physical activity to maintain good health? A pilot study', *Adapted Physical Activity Quarterly* 26(4), 307–320. https://doi.org/10.1123/apaq.26.4.307

Shields, N. & Taylor, N.F., 2010, 'A student-led progressive resistance training program increases lower limb muscle strength in adolescents with Down syndrome: A randomised controlled trial', *Journal of Physiotherapy* 56(3), 187–193. https://doi.org/10.1016/S1836-9553(10)70024-2

Shields, N., Taylor, N.F. & Dodd, K.J., 2008, 'Effects of a community-based progressive resistance training program on muscle performance and physical function in adults with Down syndrome: A randomized controlled trial', *Archives of Physical Medicine and Rehabilitation* 89(7), 1215–1220. https://doi.org/10.1016/j.apmr.2007.11.056

Shields, N., Taylor, N.F., Wee, E., Wollersheim, D., O'Shea, S.D. & Fernhall, B., 2013, 'A community-based strength training programme increases muscle strength and physical activity in young people with Down syndrome: A randomised controlled trial', *Research in Developmental Disabilities* 34(12), 4385–4394. https://doi.org/10.1016/j.ridd.2013.09.022

Singh, A.S., Paw, M.J.C.A., Bosscher, R.J. & Van Mechelen, W., 2006, 'Cross-sectional relationship between physical fitness components and functional performance in older persons living in long-term care facilities', *BMC Geriatrics* 6(1), 4–12. https://doi.org/10.1186/1471-2318-6-4

Smith, D.S., 2001, 'Health care management of adults with Down syndrome', *American Family Physician* 64(6), 1031–1039.

Temple, V.A., Walkley, J.W. & Greenway, K., 2010, 'Body mass index as an indicator of adiposity among adults with intellectual disability', *Journal of Intellectual Developmental Disability* 35(2), 116–120. https://doi.org/10.3109/13668251003694598

Terblanche, E. & Boer, P.-H., 2012, 'The functional fitness capacity of adults with Down syndrome in South Africa', *Journal of Intellectual Disability Research* 57(9), 826–836. https://doi.org/10.1111/j.1365-2788.2012.01594.x

Terblanche, E. & Boer, P.-H., 2013, 'The functional fitness capacity of adults with Down syndrome in South Africa', *Journal of Intellectual Disability Research* 57(9), 826–836. https://doi.org/10.1111/j.1365-2788.2012.01594.x

The Americans with Disabilities Act, Coverage of Contagious Diseases, 2011, 'CRS Report for Congress', viewed 06 March 2021, from https://www.everycrsreport.com/files/20110110_RS22219_2dc812560ec5a4035b2dc8db9cc398df59673d52.pdf.

Torr, J., Strydom, A., Patti, P. & Jokinen, N., 2010, 'Aging in Down syndrome: Morbidity and mortality', *Journal of Policy Practise in Intellectual Disability* 7(1), 70–81. https://doi.org/10.1111/j.1741-1130.2010.00249.x

Tsimaras, V.K. & Fotiadou, E.G., 2004, 'Effect of training on the muscle strength and dynamic balance ability of adults with Down syndrome', *Journal of Strength and Conditioning Research* 18(2), 343–347. https://doi.org/10.1519/00124278-200405000-00025

Tsimaras, V.K., Glagazoglou, P., Fotiadou, E., Christoulas, K. & Angelopoulou, N., 2003, 'Jog-walk training in cardiorespiratory fitness of adults with Down syndrome', *Perceptual and Motor Skills* 96(3), 1239–1251. https://doi.org/10.2466/pms.2003.96.3c.1239

Varela, A.M., Bettencount Sardinha, L. & Pitetti, K.H., 2001, 'Effects of an aerobic rowing training regimen in young adults with Down syndrome', *American Journal on Mental Retardation* 106(2), 135–144. https://doi.org/10.1352/0895-8017(2001)106%3C0135:EOAART%3E2.0.CO;2

Vellas, B.J., Wayne, S.J., Romero, L., Baumgartner, R.N., Rubenstein, L.Z. & Garry, P.J., 1997, 'One-leg balance is an important predictor of injurious falls in older persons', *Journal of American Geriatric Society* 45(6), 735–738. https://doi.org/10.1111/j.1532-5415.1997.tb01479.x

Villarroya, M.A., González-Agüero, A., Moros-García, T., De la Flor Marín, M., Moreno, L.A. & Casajús, J.A., 2012, 'Static standing balance in adolescents with Down syndrome', *Research in Developmental Disabilities* 33(4), 1294–1300. https://doi.org/10.1016/j.ridd.2012.02.017

Vodola, T.M., 1978, *Developmental and adapted physical education: A.C.T.I.V.E. motor ability and physical fitness norms: For normal, mentally retarded, learning disabled, and emotionally disturbed individuals*, Township of Ocean School District, Oakhurst, NJ.

Whitt-Glover, M.C., O'Neill, K.L. & Stettler, N., 2006, 'Physical activity patterns in children with and without Down syndrome', *Pediatric Rehabilitation* 9(2), 158–164. https://doi.org/10.1080/13638490500353202

Winnick, J.P. & Short, F.X., 1998, 'Project target: Criterion-referenced physical fitness standards for adolescents with disabilities final report', s.n., s.l.

Winnick, J.P. & Short, F.X., 2014, *Brockport physical fitness test manual: A health-related assessment for youngsters with disabilities*, Human Kinetics, Champaign, IL.

Wong, C.X., Sullivan, T., Sun, M.T., Mahajan, R., Pathak, R.K., Middeldorp, M. et al., 2015, 'Obesity and the risk of incident, post-operative, and post-ablation atrial fibrillation: A meta-analysis of 626,603 individuals in 51 studies', *JACC: Clinical Electrophysiology* 1(3), 139–152. https://doi.org/10.1016/j.jacep.2015.04.004

Woodward, T.W. & Best, T.M., 2000, 'The painful shoulder: part I. Clinical evaluation', *American Family Physician* 61(10), 3079–3088.

World Health Organization (WHO), 2010, *Global recommendations on physical activity for health*, World Health Organization, Geneva.

Wuang, Y. & Su, C.Y., 2012, 'Patterns of participation and enjoyment in adolescents with Down syndrome', *Research in Developmental Disabilities* 33(3), 841–848. https://doi.org/10.1016/j.ridd.2011.12.008

Wuang, Y.P. & Su, C.Y., 2009, 'Reliability and responsiveness of the Bruininks–Oseretsky Test of Motor Proficiency-Second Edition in with intellectual disability', *Research in Developmental Disabilities* 30(5), 847–855. https://doi.org/10.1016/j.ridd.2008.12.002

Yang, Q., Rasmussen, S.A. & Friedman, J.M., 2002, 'Mortality associated with Down's syndrome in the USA from 1983 to 1997: A population-based study', *The Lancet* 359(9311), 1019–1025. https://doi.org/10.1016/S0140-6736(02)08092-3

Index

www.ingramcontent.com/pod-product-compliance
Lightning Source LLC
Chambersburg PA
CBHW081347280326
41927CB00042B/3210

* 9 7 8 1 6 6 6 7 5 4 0 3 2 *